HAND PAIN
AND
IMPAIRMENT

D0064433

RENE CAILLIET, M. D.

Chairman and Professor
Department of Rehabilitative Medicine
University of Southern California School of Medicine
Los Angeles, California

F. A. DAVIS COMPANY *Philadelphia*

Also by Rene Cailliet:

LOW BACK PAIN SYNDROME

SHOULDER PAIN

NECK AND ARM PAIN

FOOT AND ANKLE PAIN

KNEE PAIN AND DISABILITY

Library of Congress Cataloging in Publication Data

Cailliet, Rene.
  Hand pain and impairment.
  Includes bibliographies and index.
  1. Hand—Diseases. 2. Hand—Wounds and injuries.
I. Title. [DNLM: 1. Hand. 2. Pain—Therapy.
WE830 C134h]
RC951.C24 1975   617'.575   75-6660
ISBN 0-8036-1617-1

Preface

While reviewing the first edition of *Hand Pain and Impairment,* it became evident to me that the text, unlike the other volumes in the *Cailliet Pain Series,* stressed impairment rather than pain. Although this revision retains the initial format, it has been expanded to include discussions of some of the many painful conditions of the hand. Many illustrations have been redrawn to more clearly aid textual explanations.

Early evaluation and adequate treatment by the primary physician are necessary to the future normal functioning of the impaired hand. Too often, because of the anatomical intricacy of the hand, early evaluation and treatment are mismanaged. Adequately informed, the primary physician—who may be a family physician, physiatrist, or internist—can reduce or avoid the need for reconstructive surgery or at least allow the patient to reach the surgeon with a salvageable hand.

Thus, the purpose of this book is to provide the nonspecialist with information that will enable him to better evaluate the impaired hand and initiate proper treatment. The text is therefore not exhaustive, and the presentation of the functional anatomy of the hand remains simplified. Although a simple explanation of a complex subject is possible, an easy understanding is not, and it is hoped that this book will facilitate that understanding.

RENE CAILLIET, M.D.

Table of Contents

Illustrations

CHAPTER 1

Functional Anatomy

The hand is a complex machine, so intricate in its construction and function that great detail must be given to the discussion of its functional anatomy. The hand is an organ of grasp as well as of fine movements. It is an organ of sensation, fine discrimination, and exquisite dexterity. The large portion of the brain that controls the hand is evidence of the intricacies of this organ.

To understand disease and damage of the hand and its treatment a basic knowledge of the normal hand is necessary. The primary role of the entire upper limb, shoulder, arm, elbow, forearm, is to place the hand in its proper position of function.

Restoration of function is the objective of treatment. Appearance, though important, is secondary. Early care is paramount as ultimate reconstructive treatment leaves much to be desired. The hand tolerates immobilization poorly so the balance between immobilization and movement is a fine line requiring good clinical judgment. Whereas the wrist can be fully immobilized for many weeks and recover complete mobility, the hand and fingers cannot survive even brief immobilization.

ANATOMY

Wrist

The wrist joint is the articulation between the forearm and the carpal bones and is known as the carpus. The radiocarpal and radioulnar joints have mobility in many planes resembling a universal joint in man-made machines. The bones forming the carpal rows and their relationship to the radius and ulna are shown in Figure 1.

The distal end of the radius is concave. It usually reaches further distally on its radial than on its ulnar side, although 60 percent have equal length. The dorsal surface is longer than the palmar (Fig. 2B). This structural configuration causes the hand to rest in a slight ulnar and palmar posture

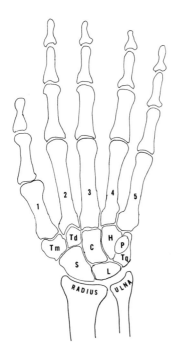

FIGURE 1. Bones of the hand. The composite of the bones of the *left* hand viewed from the palmar surface. The proximal row contains the navicular (N) (scaphoid), the lunate (L), and the triquetrum (Tq). The distal row contains the trapezium (greater multangular) (Tm), trapezoid (lesser multangular) (Td), capitate, and the hamate. The pisiform (P) is considered to be in the proximal row.

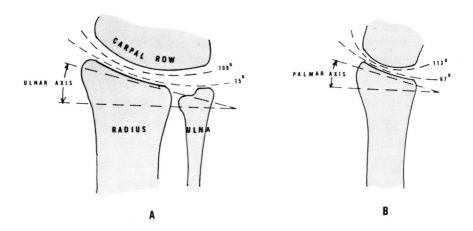

A

B

FIGURE 2. Relationship of carpal row to the radioulnar surface. The radial margin of the radius protrudes further than does the ulnar side (A). The articular surface is thus on an oblique plane. (B) The dorsal edge protrudes further than the palmar (volar) margin. The joint surfaces are incongruous; the carpal row is more convex than the opposing surface of the radius.

2

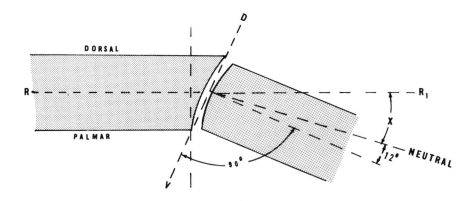

FIGURE 3. Wrist in neutral position. The *neutral* (resting) position of the wrist is slightly palmar and ulnar. Neutral is calculated as 12° of extension from plane perpendicular to the end of the radius DV and thus palmar to the axis of the radius RR₁. X is the degree of palmar flexion from the axis of the radius RR₁.

(Fig. 3). The distal end of the ulna does not articulate with any carpal bones and can be surgically removed without impairing wrist motion.

The radioulnar surface is less concave transversely than anteroposteriorly. The curvature of the proximal carpal row is greater than the opposing curve of the radioulnar surface, viewed both dorsally and laterally (Fig. 2). The discrepancy of these two curves permits greater excursion of flexion-extension than radioulnar motion. The movements of the wrist are pictured in Figure 4: 80° flexion, 70° extension, 30° ulnar abduction, and 20° radial abduction. The greater degree of flexion as compared to extension and of ulnar abduction as compared to radial is due to the angulation of the distal articular surface of the radius (see Fig. 2) and to the fact that the dorsal wrist ligaments are more slack than are the palmar ligaments.

Motion of the radiocarpal joint essentially consists of flexion-extension and transverse (radioulnar) movements (see Fig. 4.) There is *no* rotation about the longitudinal axis. Pronation and supination of the hand thus occur exclusively at the proximal radioulnar articulation in the forearm. Normal range of pronation and supination as measured with the elbow flexed is 90 degrees in either direction.

The wrist does not move in a direct plane (Fig. 5). Movement occurs along a plane between radial extension and ulnar flexion and an opposite plane of ulnar extension and radial flexion. These combined movements are related to the direction of the muscles and their tendons acting across the wrist.

All the muscles of the hand originate primarily in the forearm and pass over the wrist and carpal bones to insert into the digits. No muscle inserts

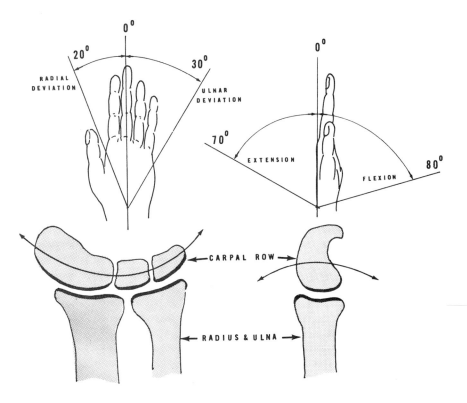

FIGURE 4. Range of wrist movement. Flexion-extension (dorsal-palmar) and lateral (radial-ulnar) are shown as an average. Neutral, as discussed in Figure 3 is not a true 0 degree. No rotation occurs about the longitudinal axis.

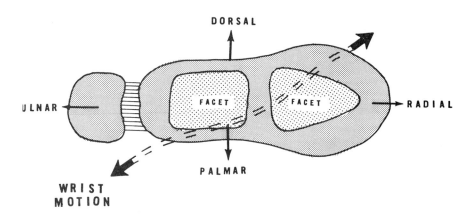

FIGURE 5. Functional movement patterns of the wrist. Wrist movements are not in one plane. All the muscles across the wrist act *obliquely*. Therefore, wrist movement is radiodorsal to ulnar-volar. This plane of wrist movement is due to antagonistic muscle group pairing—extensor carpi radialis versus flexor carpi ulnaris and the long flexors of the fingers.

into any carpal bone other than the flexor carpi ulnaris to the pisiform. They cross the radiocarpal, midcarpal, and carpometacarpal joints to attach upon the metacarpal and phalangeal bones. These tendons control the joints they traverse. As noted in Figure 5, there are two facets on the radius. The lateral facet is triangular and articulates with the scaphoid bone and the medial is cuboid and articulates with the lunate bone. A cartilage joins the distal end of the radius to the styloid of the ulna (Figs. 5 and 6). The movement of the carpal row upon the radius and the triangular ligament is that of *gliding* (see Fig. 6). As the hand flexes in a palmar direction the carpal row glides dorsally. In radial abduction of the hand, the proximal carpal row glides in an ulnar direction. To permit this gliding motion the capsule must be elastic and the ligaments sufficiently lax.

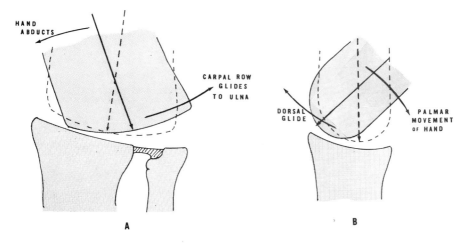

FIGURE 6. Gliding motion of the carporadial articulation. The motion between the radial surface and the proximal carpal row is that of gliding. The carpal bones glide in the opposite direction from the hand's movements. This gliding movement is permitted by capsular and ligamentous laxity.

The major functional ligaments of the wrist (Fig. 7) are essentially the longitudinal, radial, and ulnar ligaments, and the transverse and oblique ligaments located on the dorsal and palmar surfaces.

The ulnar collateral ligament arises from the styloid process of the ulna and the triangular cartilage and attaches to the pisiform. It becomes taut on radial abduction of the hand. The radial collateral ligament arises from the radial styloid process, attaches to the scaphoid and passes on to the trapezium and the first metacarpal. It becomes taut with ulnar deviation of the hand.

The transverse-oblique ligaments of the wrist on the palmar surface maintain the carpal arch. The palmar ulnar and palmar radiocarpal ligaments

5

converge at the midline to attach to the lunate and the capitate bones. This arcuate ligament is known as the ligament of Henle. The dorsal ligaments of the wrist are less symmetrical and more lax. Supination of the hand tightens the palmar ligaments, and pronation tightens the dorsal ligaments.

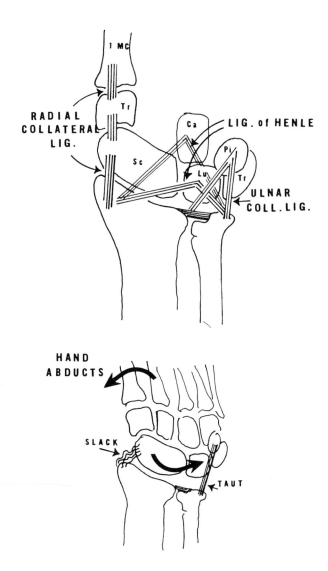

FIGURE 7. Ligaments of the wrist. The ulnar and radial collateral and the dorsal and palmar oblique ligaments support the wrist. Radial deviation of the hand tightens the ulnar collateral ligaments, and ulnar deviation tightens the radial ligaments.

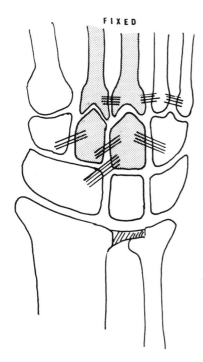

FIXED

FIGURE 8. The intracarpal ligaments. The dorsal ligaments are related. The palmar ligaments shown here are transverse in their direction radiating principally from the capitate. There are few ligaments between the proximal and distal carpal rows.

The intercarpal ligaments (Fig. 8) are placed to fortify the hand for any impact imposed upon the knuckles such as striking with a closed fist. The second and third metacarpals are fixed at their base (see metacarpal section, Chapter 1) and are immobile. The strong intercarpal ligaments strengthen the fourth and first metacarpals by their attachment to this fixed central pillar. The obliquity of these intercarpal ligaments also permits movement of the carpal bones.

Carpal Bones

The eight carpal bones are arranged in two rows. Each is cuboid with six surfaces—four surfaces covered with cartilage to articulate with the adjacent bones and two surfaces (dorsal and palmar) roughened for ligamentous attachments.

The proximal carpal row (Fig. 9) contains the scaphoid, lunate, and triquetrum. The pisiform is the fourth carpal bone in the proximal row but it is placed on the palmar surface of the triquetrum and is considered a *sesamoid* bone. The proximal carpal row articulates with the radius and the triangular cartilage to form the wrist joint.

The distal carpal row contains the os trapezium ([NA], greater multangular bone), os trapezoideum ([NA], lesser multangular bone), cap-

7

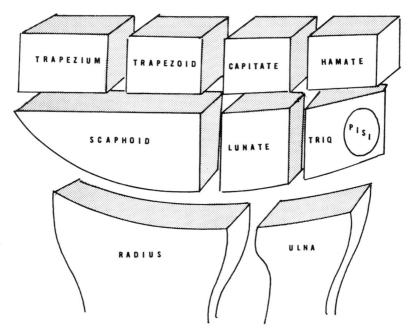

FIGURE 9. Carpal bones, schematic. The left hand is viewed from the palmar surface.

itate, and the hamate. The distal border of the proximal carpal row is concave and the proximal border convex. The trapezium and trapezoid articulate with the scaphoid, the capitate with the lunate, and the hamate with the triquetrum (see Fig. 9).

In radial abduction of the hand, the proximal row moves in an ulnar direction as does the distal row upon the proximal row (Fig. 10). The capitate glides ulnarly and approximates towards the proximal row causing a "close-packed" congruity. In ulnar deviation of the hand, the capitate moves towards the radial side and disengages from the proximal row. Of the carpal bones, the scaphoid moves the most—as much as one centimeter.

In palmar flexion and dorsal extension the distal carpi glide upon the proximal carpal row. The greatest degree of wrist-palmar flexion occurs at the radiocarpal joint, but a significant degree occurs at the intercarpal joints. In summary it can be stated that (1) palmar flexion of the wrist occurs mainly in the radiocarpal joint and secondarily in the midcarpal joints; (2) dorsiflexion (extension) occurs mostly in the midcarpal joints and secondarily in the radiocarpal joint; (3) radial deviation occurs mostly in the midcarpal joints and ulnar deviation mostly in the radiocarpal joint.

Clinically the degree of flexion-extension of the wrist can be accurately determined by placing the two hands together, palms and fingers touching,

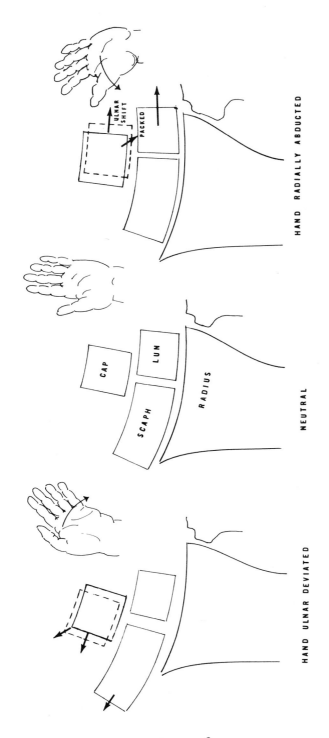

FIGURE 10. Carpal movement. When the hand moves radially, the carpal rows move in the opposite (ulnar) direction. The capitate glides ulnarly and towards the proximal row to pack tight. In ulnar movement of the hand, the opposite occurs.

9

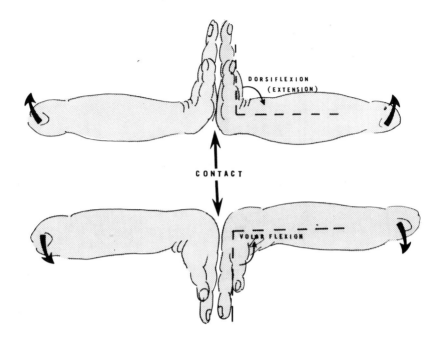

FIGURE 11. Clinical measurement of wrist flexion and extension. Wrist dorsiflexion (extension) can be estimated by placing the palms together and raising the elbows without allowing the palms to lose contact. Wrist palmar flexion can be determined by placing the backs of the hands together, fingers facing down, and then lowering the elbows until the hands begin to separate.

and raising the elbows (Fig. 11). Flexion range can be determined by placing the hands together, dorsal surface to dorsal surface, and lowering the elbows. Measurable limitation for recording requires measurement with a protractor.

Carpal Arch

The carpal bones form an arch that is concave on its palmar surface. The superficial ligament that spans this arch and maintains it, acting as a tie beam, is called the flexor retinaculum or the transverse carpal ligament (Fig. 12). This ligament is comprised of a proximal and a distal band.

The proximal band attaches from the tubercle of the navicular to the pisiform. As the pisiform is movable, this band may be relaxed. The pisiform is essentially a sesamoid bone within the tendon of the flexor carpi ulnaris. The pisiform becomes "fixed" when this tendon is taut. The proximal band of the transverse carpal ligament becomes taut when

10

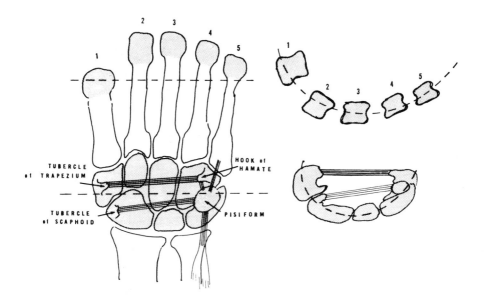

FIGURE 12. Transverse carpal ligament. Also termed the *flexor retinaculum,* this ligament bridges the arch of the carpal rows. It is formed by two bands—the proximal extending from the tubercle of the navicular to the pisiform and the distal band from the tubercle of the trapezium to the hook of the hamate.

the flexor carpi ulnaris is contracted (Fig. 13), that is when the hand is firmly held in an ulnar flexed position. The distal band of the transverse carpal ligament connects the tubercle of the trapezium to the hook of the hamate. As these are fixed points, this band is always taut.

The concavity formed by the arched carpal bones spanned by the transverse carpal ligament is termed the *carpal tunnel* (Fig. 14). This tunnel would be deep enough to permit the entrance of a finger if all its contents were removed. The tunnel contains the tendons of the flexor digitorum profundus, which lie upon the carpal bones, and their connecting ligaments. Nearer to the surface is the layer of flexor digitorum superficialis tendons. Within the canal are also found the flexor carpi radialis tendon, flexor pollicis longus tendon, and the median nerve. The transverse carpal ligament restricts the "bowing" of the long flexor tendons of the fingers when the wrist is flexed, protects the median nerve from external pressure, and is the site of origin of the thenar and hypothenar muscles.

The superficial landmarks of the structures on the palmar aspect of the wrist are shown in Figure 15. The distal skin crease of the wrist corre-

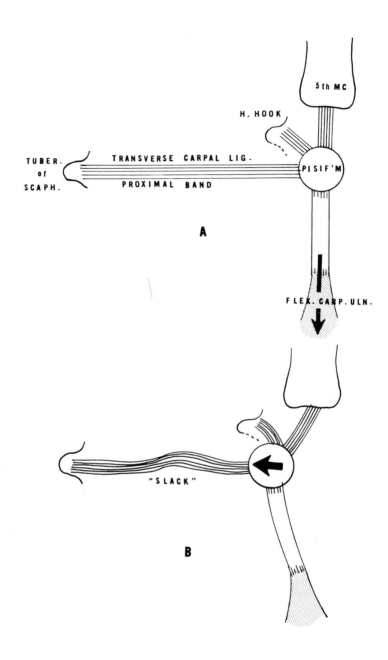

FIGURE 13. Proximal band of transverse carpal ligament. The proximal band of the transverse carpal ligament is taut or slack depending upon the tension on the pisiform by the flexor carpi ulnaris. The pisiform is a sesamoid bone within the tendon of the flexor carpi ulnaris which attaches to the base of the fifth metacarpal and the hook of the hamate. (A) The contracted muscle tenses the transverse ligament. (B) Both are slack.

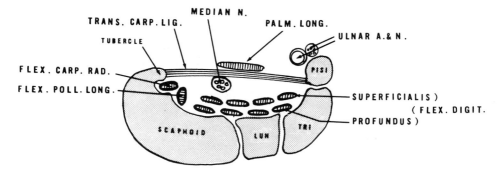

FIGURE 14. Carpal tunnel contents. The tunnel formed by the carpal bones and the spanning transverse carpal ligament contains the tendons of the long finger flexors (deep and superficial), tendons of the flexor pollicis longus and flexor carpi radialis, and the median nerve.

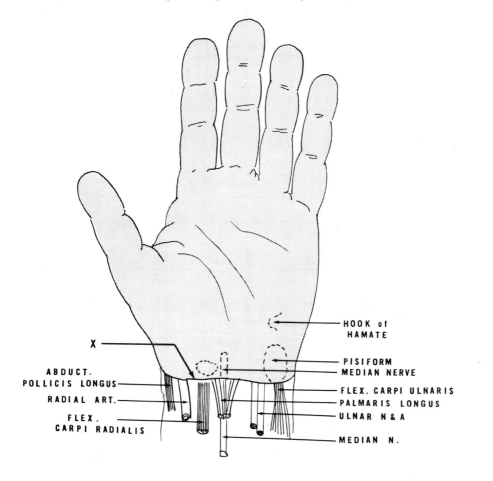

FIGURE 15. Superficial landmarks at the palmar surface of the wrist.

sponds to the proximal border of the transverse carpal ligament. The flexor carpi radialis leads to the tubercle of the scaphoid and can be palpitated when the clenched fist is flexed and radially abducted against resistance. The flexor carpi ulnaris leads to the pisiform and can be palpated when the clenched fist is flexed in an ulnar deviated direction.

The median nerve cannot be palpated at the wrist. It lies under the palmaris longus tendon which can be palpated and seen in the mid region of the wrist when the clenched fist is flexed in a midline position and against resistance.

The radial artery is palpable on the radial side between the tendon of the flexor carpi radialis and the abductor pollicis longus. The ulnar artery is palpable just to the radial side of the flexor carpi ulnaris tendon. The radial artery is readily palpable, but the ulnar artery is too deep under a thick fascia to be readily palpated.

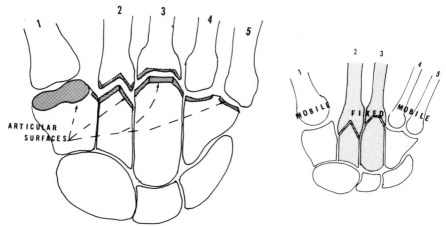

FIGURE 16. Carpometacarpal articulations. Five metacarpal bones articulate with four carpal bones. The second and the third metacarpal immobilize this segment by their numerous facets, close apposition of the planes of these facets, and the deep inset of the second metacarpal against the trapezoid and between the trapezium and the capitate. The first, fourth, and fifth metacarpals are mobile about this central fixed segment.

The Carpometacarpal Articulation

The distal border of the carpal bones is irregular. Four carpal bones articulate with five metacarpal bones. The fourth and fifth metacarpals articulate with two concave facets of the hamate (Fig. 16). The first (thumb) articulates with the saddle-shaped trapezium. The first, fourth, and fifth metacarpals have mobile joints. The second and third metacarpals form the immobile joints (Fig. 17). The second metacarpal has a gutter-shaped surface that fits over the central ridge of the trapezoid. The three

14

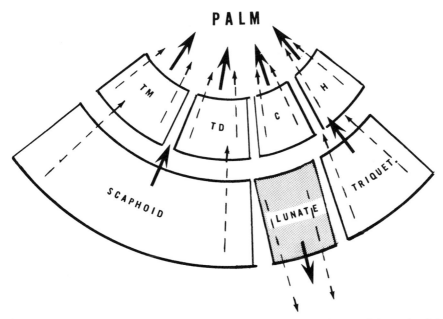

PALM

FIGURE 17. Carpal bone configuration, direction of displacement. The carpal bones by their shape form the palmar concavity and the dorsal convexity of the hand. The bones are broader on their dorsal surfaces and narrow on their palmar surface. This shape causes them to dislocate dorsally (with the exception of the lunate bone).

protruding facets of the capitate are in direct contact with the three opposing facets of the third metacarpal. There is also a small facet of the third metacarpal in contact with the base of the second metacarpal. Being so wedged both the second and third metacarpals are immobile. In the *cupping* motion of the hand, the carpometacarpal joints move about this central immobile segment. The first metacarpal articulates on the radial side and the fourth and fifth (ring and little fingers) on the ulnar side of the "fixed" segment.

Metacarpophalangeal Articulations

The distal portion of the metacarpal is covered by hyaline cartilage that extends slightly over the dorsum and around the palmar surface on a rounded surface (Fig. 18). The ends are slightly flattened. Flexion-extension (dorsal-palmar), abduction-adduction, and some rotation (pronation-supination) are possible at this joint. Flexion-extension and abduction-adduction are voluntary motions but rotation is possible only as a passive motion.

The capsule of these joints is redundant to permit motion in which the concave surface of the phalanx *glides* along the convex surface of

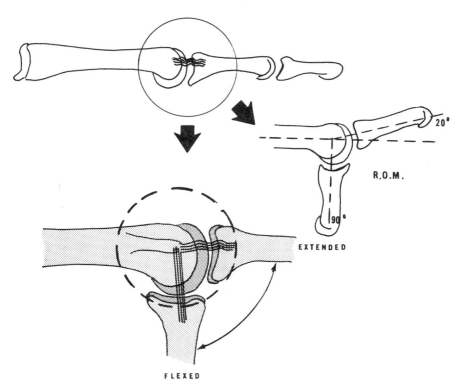

FIGURE 18. Metacarpophalangeal joints. Due to the eccentric radius of rotation about the axis of the head of the metacarpal (dotted circle), flexion of the phalanx causes the collateral ligaments to become taut. The laxity of the ligaments in extension permits some lateral motion. Range of motion is 90° flexion and 20° hyperextension.

the metacarpal. The proximal surface of the phalanx has an arc of 20° whereas the metacarpal head has a surface arc of 180°. Motion of the metacarpophalangeal joint is 90° of palmar flexion and usually 20° of hyperextension (see Fig. 18).

Abduction and adduction of the metacarpophalangeal joint is limited when the finger is flexed because the head is flattened at its distal margin and the collateral ligaments are made taut in flexion. The collateral ligaments originate from a small tubercle eccentrically located on the lateral surfaces of the head. With the finger extended, the collateral ligaments are slack and permit lateral motion. In the flexed position, the base of the phalanx seats firmly against the surface of the metacarpal surface which now is further away from the axis of rotation. The ligaments thus become taut. On the palmar aspect of the joint the condyles are also broader than at the dorsal aspect which further tightens the ligaments.

There are no ligaments on the dorsal surface of the metacarpophalangeal joints. Here the limiting tissues are the extensor tendons of the fingers. The palmar aspect of these joints is reinforced by the *palmar plates* (Fig. 19). These are fibrocartilaginous plates in which the distal portion is cartilaginous and is firmly attached to the proximal portion of the phalanx. The proximal portion of the plate is membranous and is loosely attached to the metacarpal.

The plates are held firmly against the joints by fibers of the collateral ligaments and are connected to each other by the deep transverse ligaments (Figs. 19 and 20). These plates reinforce the joint capsule and interpose between the joint surfaces and the flexor tendons that traverse the joint.

Subluxation of the metacarpophalangeal joint will often tear the plate from its metacarpal attachment. Because of the membranous portion of

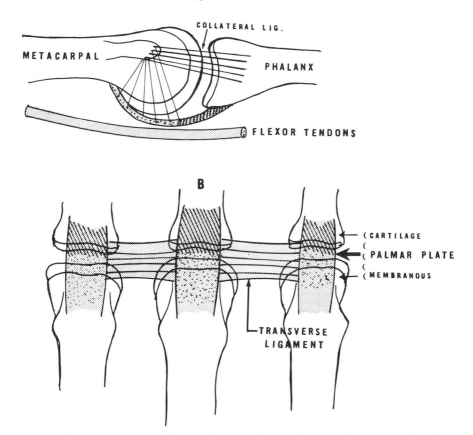

FIGURE 19. Palmar plate. A fibrocartilaginous plate replaces the ligament on the palmar surface of the joint. The cartilaginous portion is firmly attached to the phalanx (A). The proximal membranous portion is loosely attached to the metacarpal (B). The plate is firmly held to the metacarpal by fibers of the collateral ligament. (B) Palmar view shows the deep transverse ligament that connects the plates and prevents lateral motion of all the metacarpals except the thumb.

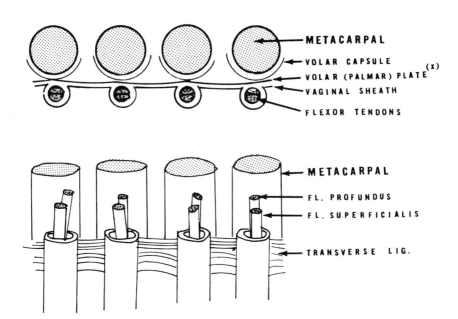

FIGURE 20. Transverse metacarpal ligament. The volar fibrocartilaginous plate reinforces the joint capsule. It also forms the dorsal portion of the vaginal ligament that forms pouches that encircle the flexor tendons as part of the tendons' gliding mechanism.

the plate, prolonged immobilization of the finger in flexion causes retraction of the membranous tissue resulting in a flexion contracture.

The palmar fibrocartilaginous plates join transversely (see Fig. 20) to form the intermetacarpal ligament. There is an outpouching of the ligament on the palmar aspect of each metacarpal which encloses the flexor tendons and forms part of the gliding apparatus of the flexor tendons. This outpouching is called the vaginal ligament.

Interphalangeal Joints

The interphalangeal joints are true hinge joints allowing only flexion and extension (Fig. 21). There are basic differences with the metacarpophalangeal joints:

1. The metacarpophalangeal joint is a ball-and-socket joint that permits abduction, adduction, and circumduction. The interphalangeal joint is a hinge joint allowing flexion and extension.
2. The articular surface configurations differ (Fig. 2B).
3. Hyperextension, at least passively, is possible at the metacarpophalangeal joint, but not at the interphalangeal joints.
4. Collateral ligaments are tight in flexion and slack in extension at

the metacarpophalangeal joints but not fully understood at the interphalangeal joints (Fig. 18).

5. At the metacarpophalangeal joints the palmar plates are connected to many mobile tissues (Fig. 19)—deep transverse ligament, tendons of the interossei and the palmar aponeurosis—whereas in the interphalangeal joints the plate is less mobile.

All these factors are implicated in the complication resulting from prolonged immobilization in an unphysiological (extended) position with resultant "stiffness" of the joints.

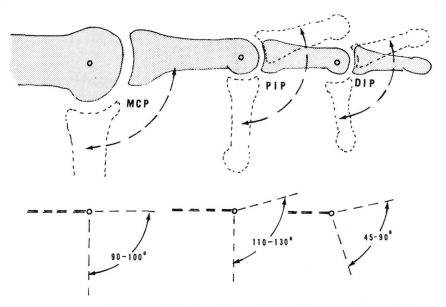

FIGURE 21. Range of motion of the interphalangeal joints. The proximal interphalangeal joint (PIP) averages 110 to 130° and the distal phalangeal joints (DIP) 45 to 90°. Both of these joints are capable of hyperextension. Further flexion is checked by the dorsal capsule. The metacarpophalangeal joint (MCP) has a range of 90 to 100°.

Muscular Control

All muscular activity of the hand, wrist, and fingers can be divided into the *extrinsic* and *intrinsic* muscle groups.

Extrinsic Muscles

All forearm muscles (except the pronator teres, supinator, and brachialis) traverse the wrist joint and the metacarpophalangeal joints. The palmar group originates from the medial condyle of the humerus and is flexor in function. The dorsal group originates from the lateral condyle of the humerus and is essentially extensor in function.

The *extensor forearm muscles* are arranged into a superficial and a deep layer with the superficial layer divided into a lateral and a posterior group. The lateral and the posterior groups of the superficial layer are separated by the extrinsic muscles of the thumb (Fig. 22).

The superficial group originates from the common extensor tendon which is attached to the lateral epicondyle area, the intermuscular septum, and along the lateral supracondylar ridge.

I. Superficial Muscles of the Extensor Forearm
   A. Lateral Group
      1. Brachioradialis crosses the cubital fossa, inserts into the base of the styloid process of the radius (see Fig. 22), flexes the elbow when the forearm is midway between pronation and supination. So, although it is in the extensor group, it acts as a flexor.
      2. Extensor carpi radialis longus originates from the ridge.
      3. Extensor carpi radialis brevis originates from the common tendon. Longus and brevis cross the "snuff box" and attach to the bases of the second and third metacarpals. They are pure *wrist* muscles.
   B. Posterior Group
      1. Extensor indicis (Fig. 23), extensor digitorum communis, extensor digiti minimi, extensor carpi ulnaris originate from the common extensor tendon. Their insertion is discussed later.
      2. Anconeus attaches from the lateral epicondyle region and crosses obliquely into the posterior surface of the ulna.

II. Deep Muscles of the Extensor Forearm
   A. Supinator
   B. Abductor pollicis longus
   C. Extensor pollicis brevis and extensor pollicis longus arise from the mid region of the ulna and radius and the interosseous membrane, proceed obliquely *over* the wrist extensors to attach to the thumb and index finger.

The flexor forearm muscles originate primarily from the medial condyle area of the humerus. This group is comprised of two categories— the *superficial* and the *deep*.

I. Superficial Group
   A. Originates as a common muscle mass from the medial epicondyle (Fig. 24).
      1. Pronator quadratus extends from the ridge of the ulna to the anterior surface of the radius, a broad band at the distal area of the forearm.

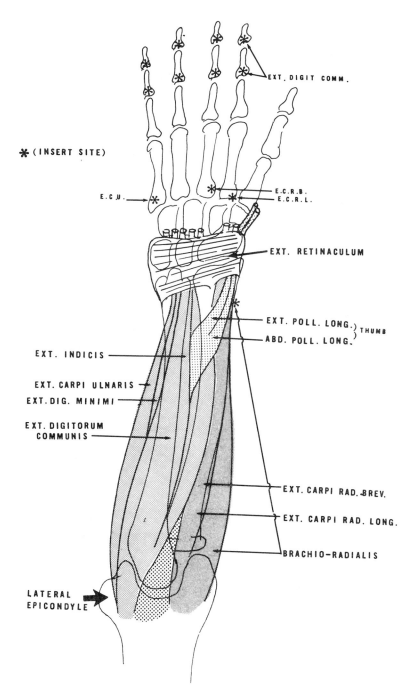

* (INSERT SITE)

EXT. DIGIT COMM.

E.C.U.

E.C.R.B.
E.C.R.L.

EXT. RETINACULUM

EXT. POLL. LONG. } THUMB
ABD. POLL. LONG.

EXT. INDICIS

EXT. CARPI ULNARIS

EXT. DIG. MINIMI

EXT. DIGITORUM COMMUNIS

EXT. CARPI RAD. BREV.

EXT. CARPI RAD. LONG.

BRACHIO-RADIALIS

LATERAL EPICONDYLE

FIGURE 22. Extensor muscles of the forearm. The origin and insertion of the extensor muscles are shown as viewed in the left arm and hand. The extensor groups comprise a superficial and deep layer which are divided by the extrinsic thumb muscles.

21

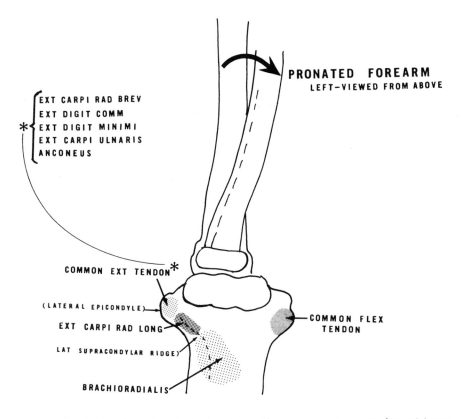

EXT CARPI RAD BREV
EXT DIGIT COMM
* { EXT DIGIT MINIMI
EXT CARPI ULNARIS
ANCONEUS

PRONATED FOREARM
LEFT-VIEWED FROM ABOVE

COMMON EXT TENDON *

(LATERAL EPICONDYLE)

EXT CARPI RAD LONG

LAT SUPRACONDYLAR RIDGE)

BRACHIORADIALIS

COMMON FLEX
TENDON

FIGURE 23. Origin of muscles about the elbow. The common extensor tendon originates from the lateral humeral epicondyle. The view presented is the pronated left elbow seen from above.

2. Flexor carpi radialis attaches to the bases of the second and third metacarpals.
3. Palmaris longus is absent in 15 percent of people.
4. Flexor carpi ulnaris attaches to the pisiform and the fifth metacarpal. The ulnar nerve enters the forearm through the two heads of this muscle.

II. Deep Layer
   A. Primarily for finger flexion (Figs. 24 and 25).
      1. Sublimis originates in the medial condyle, coronoid process of the ulna, palmar surface of the radius (see Fig. 25), and ends in four tendons inserting into the base of the second, third, fourth, and fifth middle phalanges. The sublimis separates into a superficial portion (two tendons to the middle and ring fingers) and a deep portion (tendons to the index and little fingers).

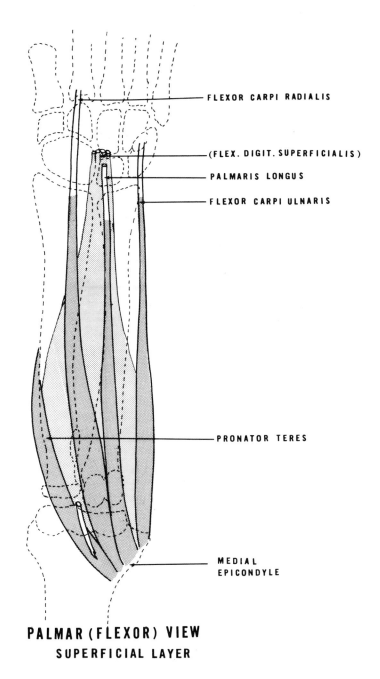

— FLEXOR CARPI RADIALIS

— (FLEX. DIGIT. SUPERFICIALIS)

— PALMARIS LONGUS

— FLEXOR CARPI ULNARIS

— PRONATOR TERES

— MEDIAL
EPICONDYLE

PALMAR (FLEXOR) VIEW
SUPERFICIAL LAYER

FIGURE 24. Palmar flexor group, superficial layer. The superficial group of flexor muscles on the palmar surface of the forearm originate from a common muscle mass at the medial epicondyle. The most medial is the pronator teres, then comes the flexor carpi radialis inserting into the base of the second and third metacarpals, the palmaris longus, and the flexor carpi ulnaris attaching to the pisiform. The flexor digitorum in the deeper layer is seen through the superficial layer.

23

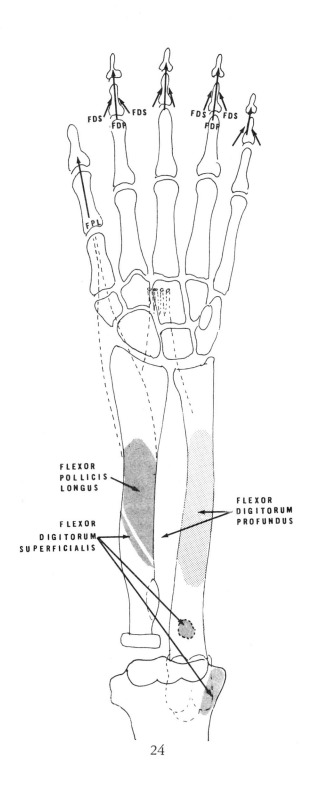

FDS FDS
FDP

FDS FDS
FDP

FPL

FLEXOR
POLLICIS
LONGUS

FLEXOR
DIGITORUM
SUPERFICIALIS

FLEXOR
DIGITORUM
PROFUNDUS

24

This is their arrangement as they pass under the transverse carpal ligament (Fig. 26).

2. Profundus (deep) common flexors arise from the ulna and interosseous membrane (see Fig. 25), cross the wrist under the carpal ligament, and attach to the distal phalanges after perforating the sublimis (superficialis) tendons (Fig. 27).

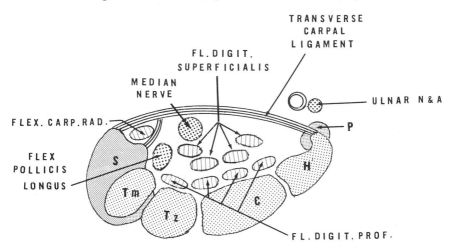

FIGURE 26. Contents of the carpal tunnel. The concave palmar surface of the carpal rows is crossed by the transverse carpal ligament. The tunnel contains the median nerve and all the flexor tendons and their sheaths. Thickening of the tendon sheaths, the carpal ligament, or deformation of the bony structure can compress the median nerve.

Lampe proposed a new terminology for muscles in 1951. Muscles are named by their locations, as in palmar forearm group and dorsal forearm group and *not* by their functions. It would better serve the purpose of functional anatomy if the palmar group (see Fig. 24) (flexor carpi radialis and ulnaris, flexor digitorum sublimis and profundus, pronator teres and quadratus) were termed *flexor pronator group.* The dorsal group (see Fig. 22) (extensor carpi radialis longus and brevis, extensor digitorum communis, indicis proprius, digiti quinti proprius, extensor pollicis brevis and longus, abductor pollicis longus and supinator) would then be termed *extensor assistant supinator group* ("assistant" because the

---

◀

FIGURE 25. Palmar flexor group, deep layer. The deep layer contains the finger flexors. The flexor digitorum sublimis originates from the medial epicondyle, the coronoid process of the ulna, and the palmar surface of the radius. It ends in four tendons attached to the base of the middle phalanges. The flexor digitorum profundus arises from the ulna and interosseous membrane and inserts into the distal phalanges. The flexor pollicis longus originates from the palmar surface of the radius and inserts into the base of the distal phalanx of the thumb.

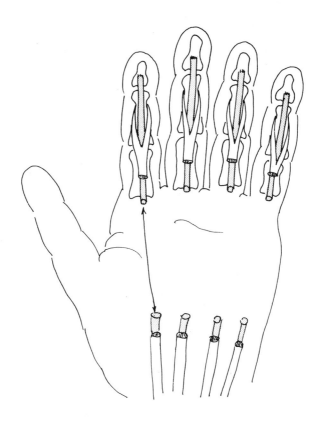

FIGURE 27. Insertion of flexor tendons. At the wrist the flexor sublimis tendons are arranged in two layers—the two inner tendons lying deep and the two outer more superficially. In their course these tendons split to allow the profundus tendons to pass through then attach to the middle phalanges of the four medial fingers. The flexor profundus tendons at the wrist are in one layer and in the same sheath as the sublimis. They pass between the split of the sublimis tendons to attach to the base of the distal phalanges.

forearm supinator *assists* the biceps). Hence, the radial nerve would be termed the *extensor assistant supinator nerve;* the ulnar nerve (which supplies the interossei) would be termed *finger spreader approximator nerve;* and the median nerve (which controls the flexor pronator group except for the flexor carpi ulnaris and the ulnar half for the flexor digitorum profundus) would be termed *flexor pronator thumb-finger approximator nerve.* All these terms are admittedly unwieldly, but functionally practical.

Tendinous Insertion into Digits

Flexor. Each profundus tendon inserts into the base of the distal phalanx (Figs. 27 and 28). The profundus is not entirely cylindrical. When it

26

passes through the superficialis it is flattened from side to side. Beyond that point, as it passes over the proximal interphalangeal joint, it is flattened from front to back. The superficialis tendon splits superficial to the proximal phalanx and forms a medial and lateral extension in a *V*-form. Each extension attaches to the lateral crest of the middle phalanx (Fig. 28). The two (medial and lateral) extensions split at the distal end of the proximal phalanx and cross over to the opposite side. This fourth of the tendon (half of the splint) passes under the profundus tendon which has passed through the perforation of the superficialis tendons.

A tubular sheath envelops the flexor tendons (Fig. 29) containing a fluid similar to synovial fluid which acts as a lubricating fluid (Fig. 30). These sheaths prevent or diminish the friction of the moving tendon against bone prominences or at points of curvature or angulation.

The palmar fascia (aponeurosis) crosses the palm and blends distally to participate in the fibrous compartments (tunnels) of the flexor tendon apparatus (Figs. 31 and 32). The palmaris longus tendon traverses the wrist in front of the transverse carpal ligament and in the palm divides

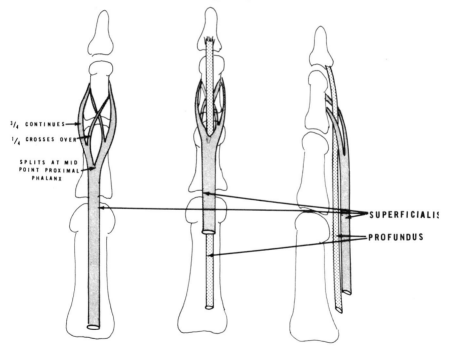

FIGURE 28. Digital flexor mechanism. The profundus tendon inserts into the entire breadth of the base of the distal phalanx, into the palmar plate, into the pulp of the finger. The sublimis tendon splits midway past the proximal phalanx. Three fourths of the fibers continue and attach to the lateral crest of the middle phalanx. One fourth crosses under the tendon of the profundus which has passed through the perforation of the sublimis tendon.

27

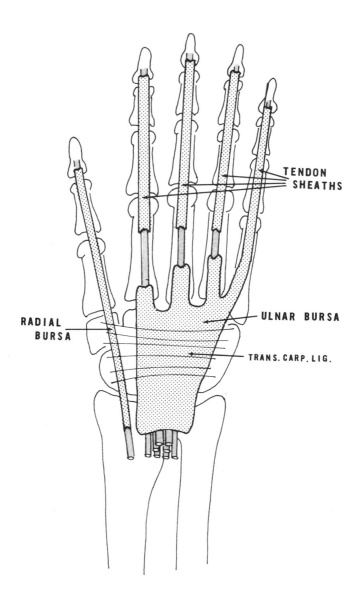

TENDON
SHEATHS

RADIAL
BURSA

ULNAR BURSA

TRANS. CARP. LIG.

FIGURE 29. Tendon sheaths and flexor bursa. The tendon sheaths of the index, middle, and ring fingers extend from the midpalmar crease to the insertion of the flexor profundus tendon into the distal phalanx. The sheath of the fifth finger continues from the ulnar bursa which is found in the palm under the transverse carpal ligament. This bursa contains all the tendons except the thumb tendon. The ulnar bursa forms three compartments—one superficial to the sublimis tendons, one between the sublimis and profundus tendons, and one under the profundus tendons. The thumb bursa (radial bursa) extends from under the transverse carpal ligament to accompany the flexor tendon to its insertion at the distal phalanx. In 15 to 20 percent of persons the fifth tendon sheath does not communicate with the ulnar bursa. Occasionally all tendon sheaths connect with the bursa.

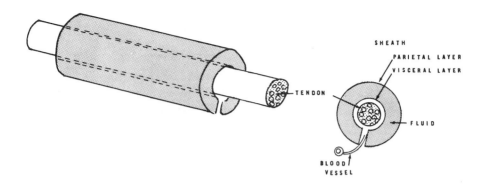

FIGURE 30. Schematic tendon sheath. The tendon sheath has two layers—the parietal and the visceral between which is a synovial fluid that acts as a lubricant. The blood vessel supplying the tendon enters by way of a fold in the sheath.

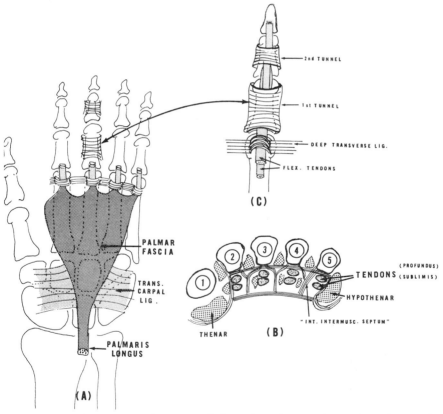

FIGURE 31. Palmar fascia. The course of the palmar fascia and its relationship to the tendons and the transverse ligaments at the metacarpophalangeal joints is shown. (A) Passage of the palmar fascia over the transverse carpal ligament and fanning out to the four medial fingers. (B) The septa arising from the fascia and descending to the metacarpals to form compartments, each containing the flexor tendons and the intrinsic muscles. (C) The fibrous tunnels that enclose the flexor tendons during their passage along the phalanges.

into four bands that pass down to the four metacarpals. At the metacarpal heads the palmar aponeurosis blends into the deep transverse carpal ligament (see Figs. 19, 20, 31, and 32). Distal to the metacarpal heads, each pair of tendons (superficialis and profundus) becomes enclosed in a fibrous sheath (see Fig. 31) which is thick and strong at the shafts of the phalanges but thin at the interphalangeal joints to permit flexibility of the fingers.

The effective length of the extrinsic finger muscles is the controlling factor in the range of combined wrist and finger movements. Neither the flexor nor the extensor muscles can allow simultaneous maximal movement of the wrist and fingers in the same direction at the same time. Thus, it is not possible to completely extend the wrist and the fingers together. The flexor digitorum superficialis and profundus and the extensor digitorum are not long enough to permit this. The most powerful finger flexion occurs with the wrist slightly extended.

Full flexion requires extensor lengthening causing a viscoelastic action (decelerating action due to elasticity) and slow viscoelastic stretching of the interossei (Fig. 33) (to be subsequently discussed). The interossei contract when the metacarpophalangeal joints flex with simultaneous interphalangeal extension. In full flexion there is an excursion of 4 to 6 cm. of the profundus and 3 to 5 cm. of the superficialis—a significant factor to consider when surgical tendon transfer is contemplated.

Intrinsic Muscles

The intrinsic muscles pertain to the muscles that originate within the hand and act upon the digits. They are comprised of the following groups.

1. The *thenar* group performs thumb function.
2. The *hypothenar* group performs little (fifth) finger function.
3. The *interossei* and the *lumbricals* perform abduction and adduction of the fingers and combine with the extensor tendons for finger extension.

The interosseus and the lumbrical muscles have a similar function, though the interossei are more consistently present and stronger than the lumbricals. The interossei, supplied by the ulnar nerve, consist of four dorsal and three palmar muscles (Figs. 34 and 35).

The dorsal interossei are bipenniform muscles that arise from adjacent sides of the opposing metacarpals and converge into lateral bands that attach to the extensor mechanism (Figs. 34, 35, 36). The first dorsal originates from two bellies between which the radial artery passes. It

30

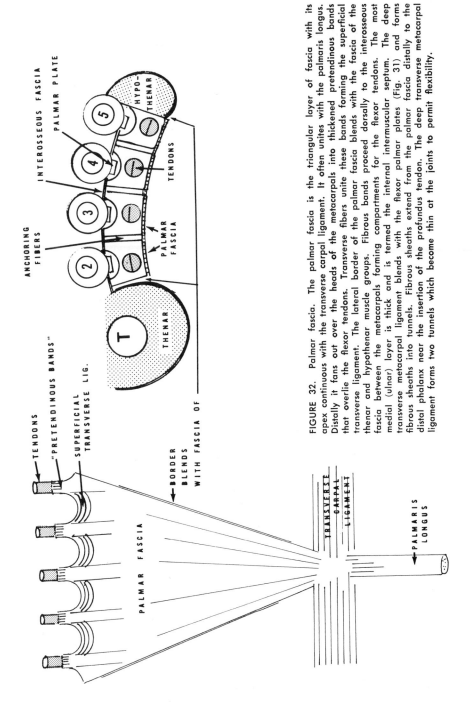

FIGURE 32. Palmar fascia. The palmar fascia is the triangular layer of fascia with its apex continuous with the transverse carpal ligament. It often unites with the palmaris longus. Distally it fans out over the heads of the metacarpals into thickened pretendinous bands that overlie the flexor tendons. Transverse fibers unite these bands forming the superficial transverse ligament. The lateral border of the palmar fascia blends with the fascia of the thenar and hypothenar muscle groups. Fibrous bands proceed dorsally to the interosseous fascia between the metacarpals forming compartments for the flexor tendons. The most medial (ulnar) layer is thick and is termed the internal intermuscular septum. The deep transverse metacarpal ligament blends with the flexor palmar plates (Fig. 31) and forms fibrous sheaths into tunnels. Fibrous sheaths extend from the palmar fascia distally to the distal phalanx near the insertion of the profundus tendon. The deep transverse metacarpal ligament forms two tunnels which become thin at the joints to permit flexibility.

31

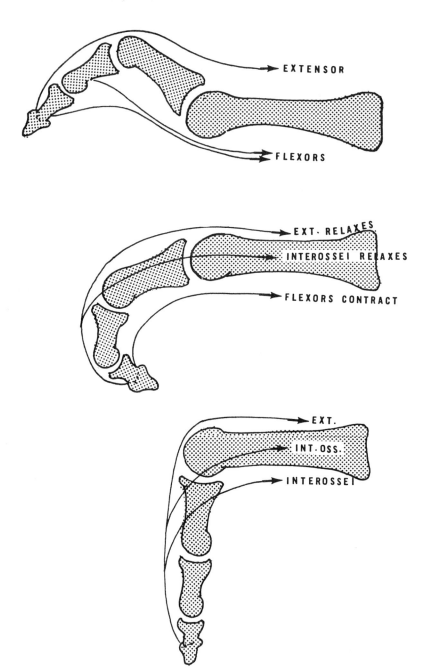

FIGURE 33. Full flexion of the digits. Normally there is action of both extensors and flexors during finger flexion. Pure action of the flexors and extensors will cause a clawing, therefore, during flexion the extensors relax their viscoelastic property as do the intrinsics (interossei). The interossei flex the metacarpophalangeal joint when the interphalangeal joints are extended.

inserts upon the radial side of the first metacarpal and produces *ab*duction of this metacarpal. It inserts upon bone 100 percent of the time (Fig. 34).

The second and third interossei insert upon the middle finger and the fourth upon the ulnar side of the ring finger. The dorsal interossei *ab*duct the index and ring finger from the midline and may move the middle finger in either a medial or lateral direction. In 50 percent of people this muscle inserts into bone and in the other 50 percent into the extensor mechanism. The interossei tendons pass dorsally to the transverse palmar ligament on their way to the extensor apparatus.

There are three palmar interossei and they function as *ad*ductors of the

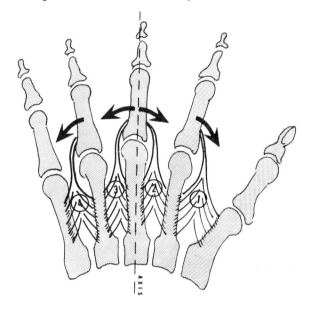

DORSAL

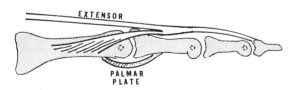

FIGURE 34. Dorsal interossei muscles. The dorsal interossei muscles with the abductor pollicis to the thumb and the abductor digiti quinti spread the fingers, that is, move them away from the axial line of the hand. The interossei arise from double muscle bellies. They pass dorsally to the transverse palmar ligaments. The first interosseous usually attaches to the bone and the others to the extensor tendon expansion.

fingers towards the middle finger (Fig. 35). The first palmar interosseus arises from the ulnar side of the second metacarpal and attaches to the extensor mechanism *on the same side.* The second interosseus originates from the radial side of the fourth metacarpal and the third from the little finger to attach to the extensor mechanism on their radial side.

There are four lumbrical muscles usually, and they arise from the radial side of the tendons of the flexor digitorum profundus and pass along the same side of the corresponding finger to attach to the extensor mechanism. Whereas the seven interossei pass behind the deep transverse ligament, the lumbricals, along with the digital nerves, pass in front (Fig. 36).

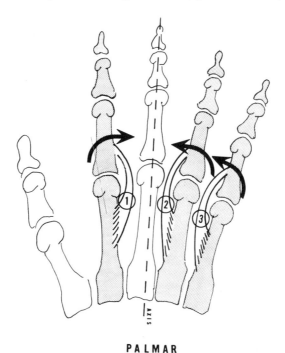

PALMAR

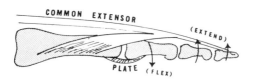

FIGURE 35. Palmar interossei, finger adductors. The thumb has its own adductor. There are only three palmar interossei arising from the second, fourth, and fifth metacarpals. The tendons pass dorsally to attach to the common extensor tendons. They adduct the fingers, flex the metacarpophalangeal joint, and extend the proximal interphalangeal joints.

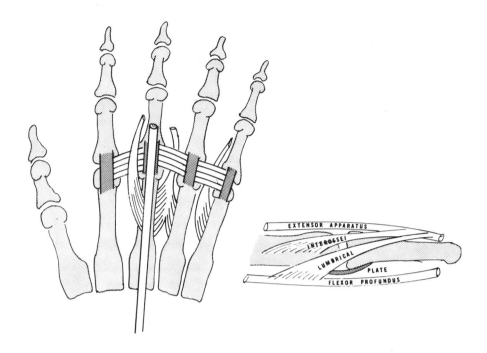

FIGURE 36. Relationship of intrinsics to the transverse ligament. The figure to the left is the palmar view of the left hand. The lumbrical originates from the flexor tendon passing dorsally to the ultimate union with the interossei into the extensor mechanism.

If the designations *palmar* and *dorsal* were eliminated from the functional concept and the interossei were regarded as *muscles lying on each side of the finger,* their function would be better understood. Each interosseus acts as a *flexor-rotator* of the proximal phalanx and extensor of the distal two phalanges. The first dorsal interosseus is a *flexor-radial deviator* and *rotator* of the metacarpophalangeal joint. It also extends the two distal joints of the index finger. The interossei of the other fingers *flex* and *rotate* these fingers and go predominantly to the ulnar side. They too are extensors of the distal two digits.

The lumbricals are predominantly interphalangeal extensors but they are not used for strength. They are richly innervated with sensory end organs and it is conceivable that they are most valuable in proprioceptive balance between the flexors and extensors in the precision action of the fingers. Long has revealed essentially *no* lumbrical activity during power grip. As shown in Figure 37, a hammering position requires a firm grip in which the fingers flex in marked *ulnar* deviation and rotation to bring them into opposition with the thenar eminence. There is also ulnar deviation of the wrist to bring the hammer handle in alignment with the forearm. Wrist motion in this plane effects the action.

In precision grip, there must be tip-to-tip opposition of the thumb and

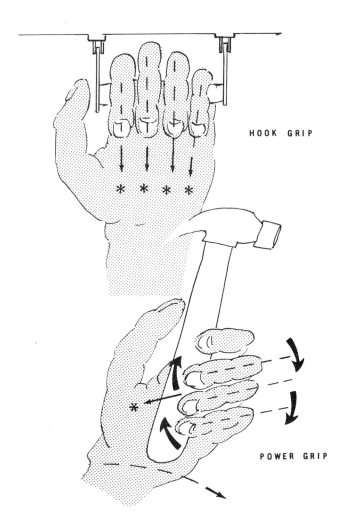

HOOK GRIP

POWER GRIP

FIGURE 37. Motion of fingers in functional movements. The hook grip is used rarely but functions to hold or lift luggage or in turning a key when the thumb presses against the side of the middle phalanx on the index finger. In the power grip, used when hammering, the fingers are flexed and rotated in ulnar deviation. The fingers flex towards the thenar eminence. The wrist also moves in an ulnar deviation, placing the hammer in alignment with the forearm. The hand grips and the wrist moves the hammer.

finger and this requires rotation and ulnar deviation of the index finger (Fig. 38). Pure anatomical finger flexion produces thumb tip to index side contact. These motions utilizing rotation and ulnar deviation are proprioceptively controlled through the action of the interossei upon the proximal phalanges and the richly innervated lumbricals.

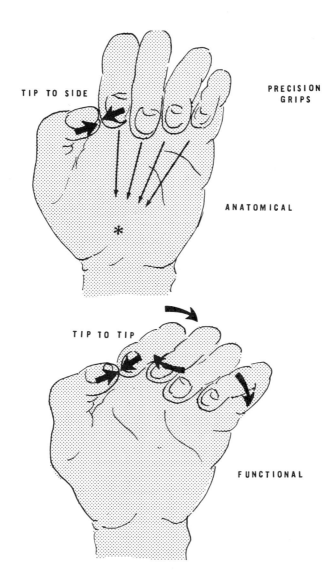

FIGURE 38. Motion of fingers in functional movements. Precision grip requires finger tip-to-tip approximation. If pure finger flexion is used the fingers flex towards the palm causing the thumb to first finger approximation to be tip-to-side. To cause tip-to-tip approximation the fingers must rotate and deviate in an ulnar direction.

Extensor Digital Mechanism

The four tendons of the extensor digitorum pass over the dorsum of the hand and under the extensor retinaculum at the wrist where they are enclosed in a synovial sheath (Fig. 39). They then proceed to the dorsum of the phalanges.

The extensor tendon splits at the distal end of the proximal phalanx and joins with the intrinsic musculature (lumbricals and interossei) to form the *extensor apparatus* of the finger (Fig. 40). Each lateral band is joined by half of an interosseous muscle tendon. More distally each is joined by the lumbrical tendon uniting on the dorsum of the proximal phalanx and attaching to the middle and distal phalanges in conjunction with the lateral bands of the extensor expansion (Fig. 41).

Without the combined action of the intrinsics, *pure* extensor digitorum action would extend the metacarpophalangeal joint and flex the interphalangeal joints. This is due to the active pull of the extensors and the passive pull of the flexor digitorum profundus (Fig. 42).

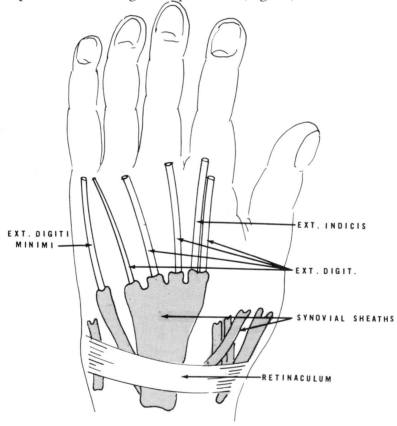

FIGURE 39. Dorsum of hand showing tendon sheaths of the extensor tendons. There are six fibro-osseous tunnels (synovial sheaths) passing under the extensor retinaculum. The extensor indicis enters the common sheath to proceed to the medial aspect of the first finger, there joining the extensor tendon. The extensor digiti quinti (proprius) has its own sheath. It is the major extensor of the little finger.

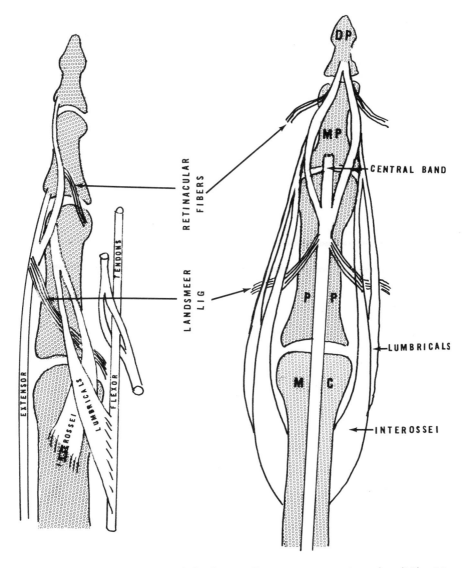

FIGURE 40. Extensor apparatus of the fingers. The extensor communis tendon divides into three components at the distal end of the proximal phalanx—a central and two lateral bands. The central band inserts into the proximal end of the middle phalanx (MP). The lateral bands pass over the lateral aspects of the proximal interphalangeal joints to converge over the middle phalanx and insert into the proximal portion of the distal phalanx (DP). A thin layer of fascia extends laterally from the extensor tendon forming a hood that encircles the interossei and lumbrical muscles. (See Figs. 45 and 46.)

Extension of the fingers requires combined action of the long extensors and the intrinsics. Extension of the proximal interphalangeal joint occurs because of combined action of three elements. The central slip of the extensor tendon (Fig. 40) inserts into the base of the middle phalanx and

39

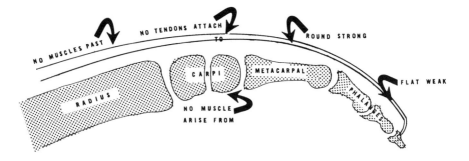

FIGURE 41. Dorsal tendon course (schematic). The course, points of attachment, and areas of attachment of the extensor tendons on the dorsum of the hand and fingers are shown.

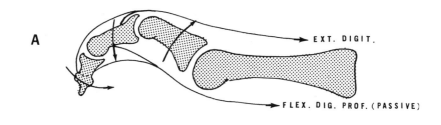

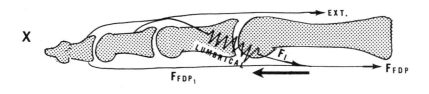

$$F_I + F_{FDP_1} = F_{FDP} \quad \therefore F_I = 0$$

FIGURE 42. Combined action of the long extensors and intrinsics. (A) Pure extensor tendon pull (without intrinsics) extends the metacarpophalangeal and flexes the proximal inter-phalangeal joints due to *passive* pull of the flexors on the distal phalanges. (X) As the extensor contracts the F_{fdp} (flexor) relaxes. The interossei F_I contracts drawing the flexor tendon forward to decrease the passive pull of the flexors. $F_I = 0$ means there is *no flexion* force at the metacarpophalangeal joint. Three muscular actions are required to extend the fingers—(1) extensor digitorum longus, (2) passive profundus, and (3) lumbrical pull upon the flexor tendon in a distal direction to relax the passive pull.

40

the two lateral bands pass to either side of the proximal interphalangeal joint to fuse distally on the middorsum of the middle phalanx to ultimately insert into the distal phalanx.

Extension of the middle phalanx is by the central slip, and the distal phalanx by the two combined slips. The length of the central and both lateral slips must be in proper alignment ("balance") to effectively extend the finger. This is why injury to or disease of these tissues creates such need for precise surgical repair. The retinacular system is *not* related to extension of the proximal joint nor, contrary to Stack's concept, significantly to extension of the distal phalanx. Many authors have shown that complete extension of the interphalangeal joints can be accomplished by the long extensors or intrinsics *alone* so long as the metacarpophalangeal joint does not hyperextend.

The lateral bands migrate dorsally as the proximal interphalangeal joint extends (Figs. 43 and 44). This is permitted by the elastic quality of the triangular ligament.

At the distal end of the metacarpal, the extensor tendon flattens to

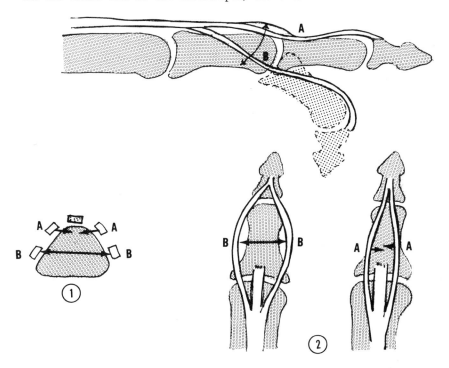

FIGURE 43. Dorsal migration of extensor lateral bands. With full extension due to the shape of the phalanx (1), and the bands becoming taut (upper figure, A), on the dorsum the bands extend approximately from (A) to (A). In (2), the left figure is the flexed phalanx, and the right figure the extended phalanx. The lateral bands migrate dorsally as the proximal interphalangeal joint extends. This is permitted by the elastic quality of the triangular ligament.

41

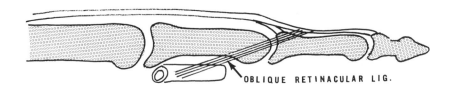

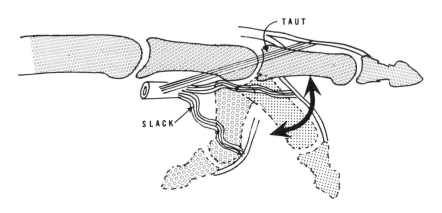

OBLIQUE RETINACULAR LIG.

TAUT

SLACK

FIGURE 44. Oblique retinacular ligament. Extension of the distal joint is aided by the tenodesis action of the retinacular ligament as the proximal joint extends. In the flexed position the ligament is slack. (See text, p. 46).

resemble a fascia and wraps around the proximal phalanx forming an expansion or a hood. This hood goes around the phalanx attaching to the transverse metacarpal ligament (Figs. 45 and 46).

The intrinsic muscles originate in the palmar aspect of the hand and pass to the dorsum of the extensor apparatus. They pass *palmar* to the joint fulcrum of the metacarpophalangeal joint and thus flex this joint (Fig. 47). They then pass *dorsal* to the fulcrum of the proximal and distal interphalangeal joints and extend these joints. As the proximal interphalangeal joint is brought into extension the retinacular ligament is placed under tension and extends the distal interphalangeal joints (tenodesis action) (Fig. 44). The two joints move in concert and always at the same angle (Stack). The oblique retinacular ligament extends the distal joint from 90 to 45° and the lateral bands from 45° to full extension (0°). This concept has been refuted by Harris and Rutledge, who sectioned the retinacular ligament and found no loss of extension from 70 to 90°. It was their conclusion that active extension of the distal phalanx is therefore caused entirely by the lateral bands, with the retinacular ligaments acting as stabilizers by maintaining the central position of the extensor tendon. Hood action appears to be the most effective extensor of the proximal phalanx.

During forceful gripping, primarily a function of the *extrinsic flexor*,

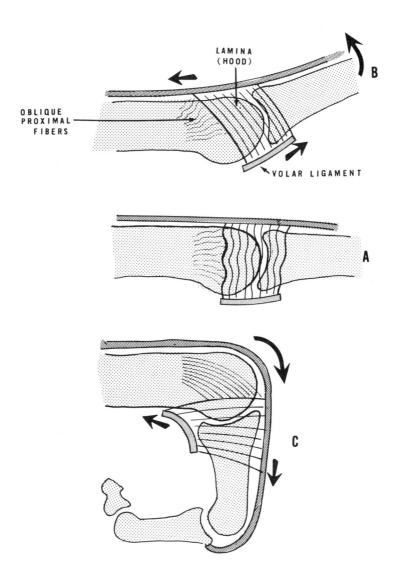

LAMINA
(HOOD)

OBLIQUE
PROXIMAL
FIBERS

VOLAR LIGAMENT

B

A

C

FIGURE 45. Extensor of metacarpophalangeal joint. Action of the transverse lamina (hood) upon the phalanges. (A) The finger is in neutral position. The transverse lamina is relaxed permitting the digits to be moved laterally by the interossei. In this position the collateral ligaments are also relaxed (Fig. 18). (B) The finger is shown in hyperextended position. The extensor tendon displaces the lamina proximally. As the proximal phalanx extends, the volar ligament is moved distally. The lamina becomes taut helping to extend the proximal phalanx. The oblique proximal fibers that attach from the extensor tendon and the lamina to the metacarpal neck periosteum are slackened. (C) In full flexion the extensor tendon moves distally causing the fibers of the lamina and the oblique proximal fibers to become taut. The flexor tendon moves the volar ligament proximally. This motion stabilizes the joint and fixes the extensor tendon. The oblique fibers limit the extent of motion of the extensor tendon.

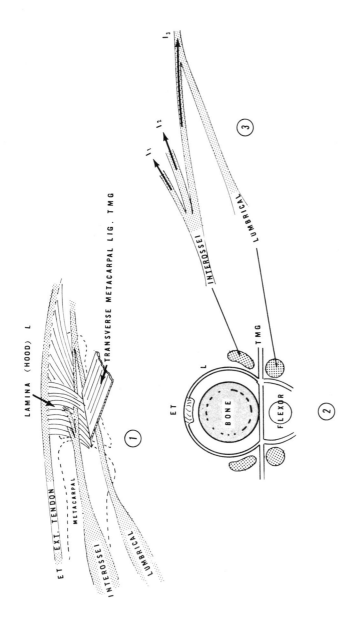

FIGURE 46. Extensor expansion detailed, the hood. (1) as the extensor tendon passes the end of the metacarpal, it expands into a flattened tissue resembling fascia and wraps around the proximal phalanx forming a hood. The interosseous muscle tendon divides into three slips—I_1 inserting into the bone which allows lateral finger motion (abduction-adduction), I_2 inserts into the lamina thus stabilizing the extensor tendon, and I_3 proceeds to unite with the lumbrical tendon (which has passed under the transverse metacarpal ligament) to merge with the lateral bands of the extensor expansion. (2) Graphic cross section showing the two intrinsic muscles, the transverse ligament (TMG), the extensor tendon (ET), and the palmar longitudinal septum that encircles the flexor tendons. (3) Graphic view of the distribution of the interossei and lumbrical tendons as noted in (1).

44

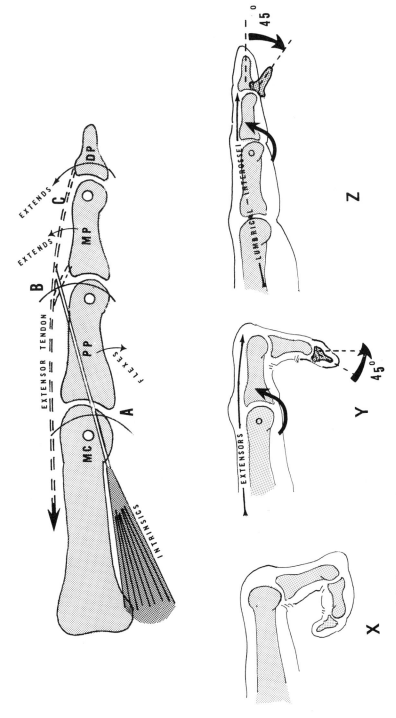

FIGURE 47. Action of the long extensors and intrinsics. (A) The intrinsics (interossei and lumbricals) lie on the palmar side of the metacarpophalangeal joint and thus flex this joint. (B) They pass to the dorsum of the fulcrum of the proximal interphalangeal joint and extend this joint. (C) The intrinsics attach to the extensors which in turn attach to the distal phalanx extending this joint (distal interphalangeal). The interossei and lumbricals cannot extend the interphalangeal joints (B) and (C) unless the metacarpophalangeal joint (A) is stabilized by the extensor tendon. (X) Depicts flexed finger. (Y) Flexing proximal interphalangeal joint extends distal phalanx 45° by means of ligamentous action. (Z) Extending the proximal joint permits flexion of the interphalangeal joint 45°, indicating laxity of Landmeer's ligament.

45

an unusual amount of extensor activity is noted by electromyogram. As the extensors should primarily open the grip, it is postulated that the extensor activity prevents palmar subluxation of the metacarpophalangeal joint.

The extensor tendons of the index and little fingers are joined on their medial side at the metacarpophalangeal joints with isolated tendons—extensor indicis to the index finger and the extensor digiti minimi to the little finger. The extensor indicis enters the same fibrous tunnel as the common tendons, but the extensor digiti minimi has its own sheath. The extensor digitorum tendon to the fifth finger is often a frail slip, so the digiti minimi is the main extensor of the little finger.

Intrinsic Muscles of the Thenar and Hypothenar Groups

The thenar muscles move the thumb. They include the following:

1. Abductor pollicis brevis arises from the tubercle of the scaphoid ridge of the trapezium and the transverse carpal ligament. It inserts into the radial aspect of the base of the proximal phalanx of the thumb.
2. Flexor pollicis brevis arises from the ridge of the trapezium and the transverse carpal ligament. It inserts into the radial side of the base of the proximal phalanx, sends an insertion into the extensor expansion, has a deep portion that originates from the base of the metacarpal, and inserts into the ulnar sesamoid.
3. Opponens pollicis lies beneath (1) and (2) and arises from the ridge of the trapezium and the transverse carpal ligament. It inserts along the entire margin of the first metacarpal.
4. Adductor pollicis has a *transverse* portion that originates from the third metacarpal and inserts into the ulnar sesamoid of the thumb. Its *oblique* portion arises from the bases of the second and third metacarpals and the capitate bone. It inserts into the ulnar sesamoid.

The hypothenar muscles move the little finger and include the following:

1. Abductor digiti minimi forms the ulnar convex surface of the hand. It originates from the pisiform bone and inserts into the ulnar aspect of the base of the proximal phalanx of the fifth finger (Fig. 48).
2. Flexor digiti minimi arises from the hook of the hamate and the transverse carpal ligament. It inserts into the ulnar side of the base of the proximal phalanx of the little finger.
3. Opponens digiti minimi lies under (1) and (2) and arises from the hook of the hamate and the transverse carpal ligament. It inserts along the ulnar side of the fifth metacarpal.

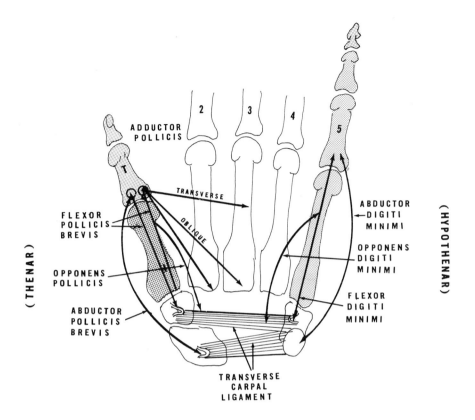

FIGURE 48. Muscles of the thenar and hypothenar regions (schematic). The muscles moving the thumb and little finger are shown. Only the intrinsic muscles are shown.

4. Palmaris brevis (not shown in Fig. 49) arises from the transverse carpal ligament. It inserts into the skin of the hand on the ulnar side.

The movements of the thumb and little finger occur in numerous planes which require definition (see Fig. 49). The thumb movement is that of the metacarpal upon the saddle-shaped joint of the trapezium (Fig. 50). Opposition of the thumb is a combination of all motions; it begins as extension to abduction, proceeds into flexion, then into adduction. The muscles of the thumb which contract during firm opposition differ from those in soft opposition. Firm opposition occurs primarily from the flexor pollicis brevis.

Nerve Control of the Hand

The Median Nerve. The median nerve in its passage along the forearm supplies the following muscles.

1. Pronator teres (C_6, C_7) pronates the forearm.

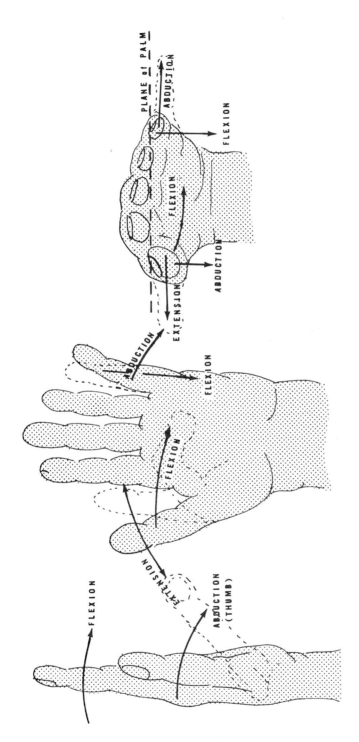

FIGURE 49. Definition of movement. Thumb: (1) Extension consists of movement away from the radial side of the index finger in the plane of the palm. (2) Abduction is movement away from the palm in a plane 90° to that of the plane of the palm. (3) Flexion is made up of movement in a plane parallel to that of the palm so as to sweep the ulnar side of the thumb across the palm. Little finger: (1) Extension involves full extension of all the joints of the little finger. (2) Abduction consists of movement away from the ring finger in the plane of the palm. (3) Flexion is 90° flexion of the finger at the metacarpophalangeal joints with the interphalangeal joints in extension.

48

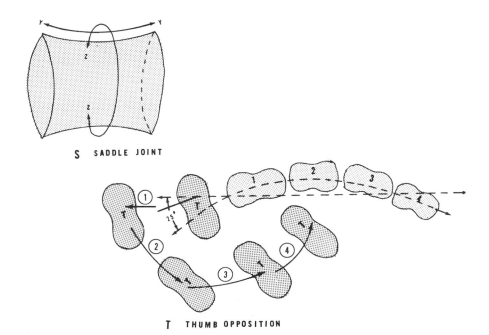

S SADDLE JOINT

T THUMB OPPOSITION

FIGURE 50. Thumb: metacarpal joint. The trapezium first metacarpal joint (thumb) is a saddle joint in which two planes of motion that are tangential to each other are possible (S). The plane of the resting thumb is 25° to the plane of the other metacarpals. Opposition of the thumb is a combination of consecutive motions: (1) extension in the plane of the palm, (2) into abduction into the palm, (3) flexion of the metacarpophalangeal joint, (4) with simultaneous adduction to the opposing finger.

2. Flexor carpi radialis (C_6, C_7, C_8) flexes the wrist in a radial direction.
3. Palmaris longus flexes the wrist.
4. Flexor digitorum superficialis (C_7, C_8, T_1) flexes the proximal interphalangeal joint.
5. Flexor digitorum profundus (C_8, T_1) flexes the distal phalanx of the index (second) and long (third) fingers.
6. Flexor pollicis longus (C_8, T_1) flexes the distal digit of the thumb.

The nerve passes under the transverse carpal ligament at the wrist and enters the palm of the hand where it splits into two branches. The lateral (motor) branch goes to the abductor pollicis brevis, the opponens, the flexor pollicis brevis, and the first and second lumbricals. These make up the small muscles of the thumb forming the thenar eminence (Fig. 51). The median (sensory) branch passes into the second and third web spaces.

The function of the median nerve is emphasized by the impairment that results from a complete median nerve paralysis.

1. Inability to *oppose* the thumb.

49

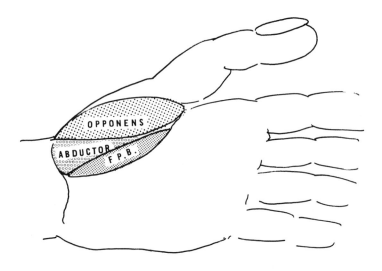

FIGURE 51. Musculature of the thenar eminence. The three muscles of the thenar eminence, innervated by the median nerve, are so positioned. This anatomical arrangement
facilitates the insertion of E.M.G. needles during diagnostic examination.

2. Inability to make a complete fist.

3. Atrophy of the thenar eminence.

The usual sensory distribution of the median nerve is shown in Figure 52. Paresis of the thenar muscles is difficult to evaluate clinically or to differentiate because of the possible substitution movements that mimic the requested motion. The opponens pollicis brings the tip of the thumb to the tip of the little finger with the thumb nail parallel to the plane of the palm. The combined action of the flexor pollicis brevis and the adductor pollicis (supplied by the ulnar nerve) will also oppose the thumb. The *abductor* pollicis brevis elevates the thumb away from the palm at a right angle to the plane of the palm (see Fig. 49). But this movement is an unreliable clinical evaluation.

Whereas 95 percent of people have the usual median innervation, the remaining 5 percent have a variation between median and ulnar motor supply. In 1 percent either the median *or* the ulnar nerve supplies *all* the muscles of the hand with the aberration occurring usually at the elbow region or in the forearm. These anomalies can be verified by electromyographic correlation with percutaneous nerve stimulation.

A partial median hand has been described in which the median supply to the first dorsal interosseus is the most common deviation. Many combinations are obviously possible.

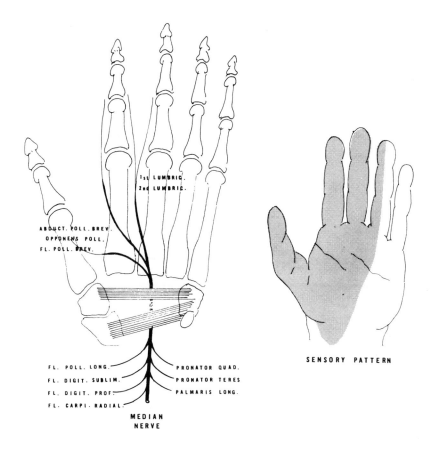

Labels on figure:
1st LUMBRIC.
2nd LUMBRIC.

ABDUCT. POLL. BREV.
OPPONENS POLL.
FL. POLL. BREV.

FL. POLL. LONG.
FL. DIGIT. SUBLIM.
FL. DIGIT. PROF.
FL. CARPI. RADIAL.

PRONATOR QUAD.
PRONATOR TERES
PALMARIS LONG.

SENSORY PATTERN

MEDIAN
NERVE

FIGURE 52. Median nerve. The motor branches of the median nerve are shown in the left figure and the right figure shows the sensory pattern of the median nerve.

Ulnar Nerve. The ulnar nerve in its passage along the forearm supplies the following muscles (see Fig. 53):

1. Flexor carpi ulnaris (C_8, T_1) flexes the wrist in an ulnar direction. It flexes the wrist when the little finger abducts.
2. Flexor digitorum profundus (C_8, T_1) flexes the distal digit of the little finger and usually the ring finger. The latter is often innervated by the median nerve.

In the hand, the ulnar nerve supplies the following:

1. Abductor digiti minimi abducts the little finger in the plane of the palm.
2. Opponens digiti minimi opposes the little finger towards the thumb.
3. Adductor pollicis (C_8, T_1) adducts the thumb in the plane of the palm.
4. Palmar interossei (C_8, T_1) adduct the fingers towards the midline.
5. Dorsal interossei (C_8, T_1) abduct all the fingers away from the midline.

51

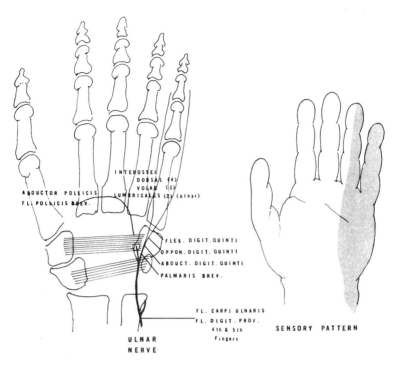

FIGURE 53. Ulnar nerve. Shows the motor and sensory distribution of the ulnar nerve.

Severance of the ulnar nerve at the elbow causes the following:

1. Flexion deformity of the fourth and fifth fingers (paralysis of the lumbrical muscles).
2. Hypothenar eminence atrophy.
3. Atrophy of interossei.
4. Atrophy of web between the thumb and index finger (first dorsal interosseus and adductor pollicis).

There is weakness of wrist flexion in the ulnar direction, weakness of flexion of the distal digit of the little finger. When the nerve is interrupted at the wrist there is weakness in abducting and adducting the fingers.

Ulnar loss at the wrist causes loss of adductor sweep of the thumb. Normally the thumb, as it adducts, sweeps across the heads of the meta-carpals and maintains continuous contact with the palm. Ulnar paralysis also causes a *positive Froment's sign* which implies the patient's inability to grasp a piece of paper between the thumb and the radial side of the palm. Abduction of the index finger in the palmar plane is lost. Care must be exercised in this determination as this motion can be mimicked by the extensor digitorum.

An innervation anomaly is possible creating an *all ulnar hand* in which all the small muscles of the hand receive their supply from the ulnar nerve. Variations in different combinations are also possible.

In summary it can be stated that the median nerve supplies opposition of the thumb to the index and middle fingers and is essential for *precision grip.* The ulnar nerve is essential for *power grip* as it controls the ulnar deviation of the fingers (see Fig. 37) through the action of the interossei and the hypothenar muscles and the two flexor profundi on the ulnar side. The ulnar nerve also supplies the forceful wrist flexor (flexor carpi ulnaris). A skilled profession could still be practiced by a person with an ulnar nerve palsy but heavy manual labor could not.

Radial Nerve. The radial nerve enters the forearm just anterior to the lateral epicondyle of the humerus and divides into both a superficial and a deep branch. The superficial branch descends to the wrist and supplies the sensation to the dorsum of the hand (Fig. 54). The deep branch

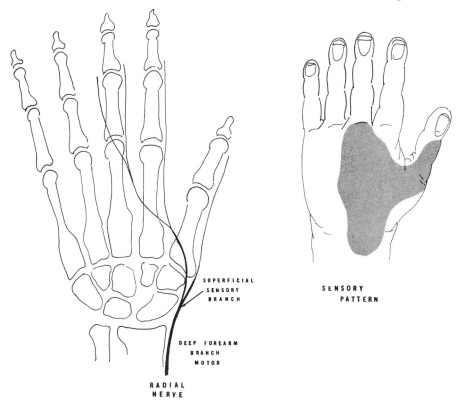

SUPERFICIAL
SENSORY
BRANCH

SENSORY
PATTERN

DEEP FOREARM
BRANCH
MOTOR

RADIAL
NERVE

FIGURE 54. Radial nerve. The sensory pattern is shown on the right, the motor distribution on the left. Above the elbow, the nerve supplies the elbow extensor (triceps), flexion (brachioradialis), and the extensor carpi radialis. Below the elbow the nerve supplies extension of the wrist in the ulnar deviation, extension of the fingers, and extension of the distal phalanx of the thumb and index finger.

passes down the forearm as the dorsal interosseous nerve and supplies the extensors of the thumb and fingers. In the upper arm it supplies the extensor carpi radialis, the triceps, and the brachioradialis.

In the forearm the radial nerve supplies the following:

1. Supinator brevis supinates the forearm.
2. Extensor carpi ulnaris extends the wrist in an ulnar direction.
3. Extensor digitorum extends the metacarpophalangeal joints.
4. Abductor pollicis longus abducts the thumb in the plane of the palm.
5. Extensor pollicis longus extends the distal digit of the thumb.
6. Extensor pollicis brevis extends the proximal phalanx of the thumb.

Complete radial nerve palsy below the triceps motor branch, in its auxiliary course, causes the following:

1. Wrist drop.
2. Inability to extend metacarpophalangeal joints of the fingers. The interphalangeal joints are supplied by the ulnar innervated intrinsics and can extend.
3. Inability to extend the distal joint of the thumb. The distal interphalangeal joint can be extended by the flexor pollicis brevis and the abductor pollicis (see Fig. 46).

If the radial nerve is interrupted in the forearm below the elbow there is inability to extend the thumb and fingers but *no* wrist drop. Attempted wrist extension deviates radially due to the action of the extensor carpi radialis and the loss of the extensor carpi ulnaris. If the lesion is below the nerve to the extensor carpi radialis, the hand extends in radial deviation but the fingers do not extend. Distal to the extensor digitorum nerve all functions remain except the thumb extensor. Injury to the nerve at the dorsum of the wrist merely causes sensory loss (Fig. 54).

Blood Supply

The radial artery becomes superficial at the wrist, winds around the styloid process of the radius, and passes under the tendons of the abductor pollicis longus and the extensor pollicis longus and brevis. It then passes through the two heads of the first dorsal interosseous muscle to enter the palm (Fig. 52). In the palm it crosses the metacarpals forming the

---

FIGURE 55. Arterial supply of the hand. The radial and the ulnar arteries meet in a deep and a superficial volar arch. At the wrist they both give off a dorsal branch that forms a dorsal arch.

◀

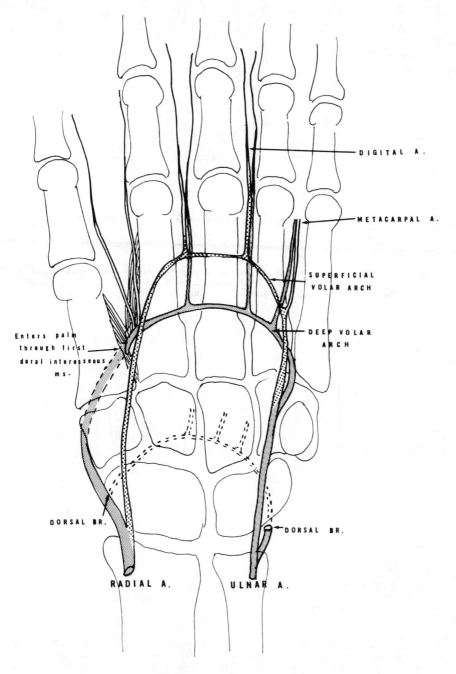

DIGITAL A.

METACARPAL A.

SUPERFICIAL
VOLAR ARCH

DEEP VOLAR
ARCH

Enters palm
through first
doral interosseous
ms.

DORSAL BR.

DORSAL BR.

RADIAL A.

ULNAR A.

PALMAR VIEW

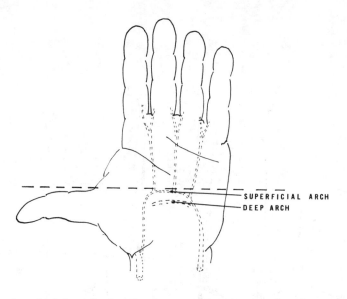

FIGURE 56. Superficial location of the palmar arterial arches. A line drawn across the palm at the distal level border of the fully extended thumb marks the site of the superficial arterial palmar arch. The deep arch is one finger breadth proximal to the superficial arch.

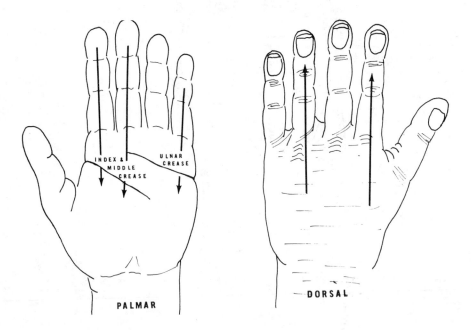

FIGURE 57. Skin creases. Creases allow the skin to fold during flexion and to extend during finger and wrist extension. The distal medial crease folds when the ulnar half of the hand flexes. The radial proximal crease folds during flexion of the middle and index fingers. The creases of the digits are attached to the tendon sheaths and permit flexion. All creases on the dorsum of the hand lie 90° to the line of pull to permit extension during the making of a fist. The loose skin is attached near the finger nail at the distal phalanx.

56

deep volar arch and unites with the ulnar artery (deep branch) (see Fig. 52).

At the wrist the radial artery gives off a superficial branch that passes over the thenar mass of muscles and runs between the palmar fascia and the flexor digitorum superficialis tendons to form the superficial volar arch. It joins the ulnar artery that has just crossed over the transverse carpal ligament. The ulnar artery divides into its deep volar branch just distal to the pisiform bone.

From the superficial arch the digital arteries arise to the index, middle, ring, and little fingers. The arterial supply to the thumb and the branch to the index finger arise from the deep radial arch at its point of emergence through the first dorsal interosseous muscle. The metacarpal arteries originate from the deep volar arch. The dorsum of the hand is supplied by an arch formed by union of the dorsal branch of the radial and the ulnar arteries.

Skin

One quarter of all Pacinian nerve endings (touch sensations) are found in the skin of the hand. Incisions and repairs of injuries must take this into consideration and also realize the detrimental effect of suturing without attention to normal creases.

Palmar creases occur during flexion of the fingers and are connected to underlying skeletal components by fascial connections. Incision in the palm should be made *parallel to but not in the creases.* The palmar skin of the digits is normally attached directly to the tendon sheaths to prevent bunching during flexion of the fingers. The skin of the dorsum of the hand is loose and wrinkled to allow elongation and free movement during finger flexion. The dorsal wrinkles are thus at right angles to the line of pull (Fig. 57).

BIBLIOGRAPHY

Backhouse, K. M.: Functional anatomy of the hand. Physiotherapy. 54:114, 1968.

Barnett, C. H., Davies, D. V., and MacConaill, M. A.: Synovial Joints: Their Structure and Mechanics. Charles C Thomas, Publisher, Springfield, Ill., 1961.

Bradley, K. C., and Sunderland, S.: The range of movement at the wrist joint. Anat. Rec. 116:139, 1953.

Byrne, J. J.: The Hand: Its Anatomy and Diseases. Charles C Thomas, Publisher, Springfield, Ill., 1959.

Flatt, A. E.: The Care of Minor Hand Injuries, ed. 2. C. V. Mosby Co., St. Louis, 1963.

Forrest, W. J., and Basmajian, J. W.: Function of human thenar and hypothenar muscles. An electromyographic study of twenty-five hands. J. Bone Joint Surg. 47-A:1585, 1965.

Grant, J. C. Boileau: A Method of Anatomy, ed. 5. Williams & Wilkins Company, Baltimore, 1952.

Haymaker, W., and Woodhall, B.: Peripheral Nerve Injuries: Principles of Diagnosis. W. B. Saunders Company, Philadelphia, 1953.

Hollinghead, W. H.: Functional Anatomy of the Limbs and Back. W. B. Saunders Company, Philadelphia, 1952.

Hulten, O.: Uber anatomische Variationen der Handgelenkknochen. Acta Radiol. 9:155, 1928.

Kaplan, E. B.: Functional and Surgical Anatomy of the Hand, ed. 1. J. B. Lippincott Company, Philadelphia, 1953.

Kuczynski, K.: The proximal interphalangeal joint. J. Bone Joint Surg. 50-B:656, 1968.

Lampe, E. W.: Surgical anatomy of the hand. Clin. Sympos. 9, 1957, *from* Surgical anatomy of the hand. CIBA edition, 1951.

Long, C.: Highland View Hospital Report, Nov. 1968, III., No. 1. Ampersand Research Group Medical Engineering, Cleveland, Ohio.

Marinacci, A. O.: Applied Electromyography. Lea & Febiger, Philadelphia, 1968.

Murphy, A. F., and Stark, H. H.: Closed dislocation of the metacarpophalangeal joint of the index finger. J. Bone Joint Surg. 49-A:1579, 1967.

Napier, J.: The Prehensile movements of the human hand. J. Bone Joint Surg. 38-B:902, 1956.

Oester, Y. T., and Mayer, J. H.: Motor Examination of the Peripheral Nerve Injuries. Charles C Thomas, Publisher, Springfield, Ill., 1960.

Papathanassiou, B. T.: Variants of the motor branch of the median nerve in the hand. J. Bone Joint Surg. 50-B:156, 1968.

Verdan, C. E.: Half a century of flexor tendon surgery. J. Bone Joint Surg. 54-A:472, 1972.

Zancolli, E.: Structural and Dynamic Bases of Hand Surgery. J. B. Lippincott Company, Philadelphia, 1968.

CHAPTER 2

Nerve

Nerve impairment in the hand probably constitutes its major disability. The hand can function adequately with motor deficit but is practically useless as a skillful tool with loss of high quality sensation. Both proprioceptive and fine tactile sensation are necessary for skilled motor activities as well as for fine tactile discrimination.

Nerve impairment can be divided into nerve severance and nerve compression. Knowledge of anatomical distribution is essential for correct diagnosis. The three major nerves serving the hand, the median, ulnar, and radial, have both motor and sensory functions.

NERVE SEVERANCE

Following an injury in which a nerve section or tendon division may have occurred, as accurate a diagnosis as possible must be made before anesthesia is administered and surgery begun. Exploratory surgery to a hand for nerve or tendon section must never be undertaken as an initial procedure. If there is an apparent nerve interruption but the cause and extent are not immediately known, carefully documented tests must be made and recorded. Many nerve lesions seen immediately after injury may have transient impairment due to edema or a contusion with ultimate recovery.

Sensory testing must follow a pattern established by the examiner which can be interpreted by subsequent examiners with similar evaluations. Initially, the patient should be asked to outline the area and indicate if the sensation is gone or changed. Sensory tests attempt to map the skin sensory areas as shown in Figure 58. This will crudely establish gross sensation in one of the major nerves supplying the hand. Most tests evaluate response to pain, light touch, and temperature which are considered to be protective sensations. These gross sensations do not evaluate functional loss.

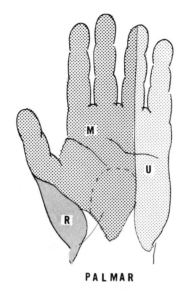 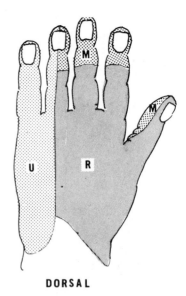

PALMAR   DORSAL

FIGURE 58. Sensory map of peripheral nerves. The schematic areas of sensory innervation of the median nerve (M), the radial nerve (R), and the ulnar (U) are shown. The dorsum of the hand is variable and the radial nerve may have *no* sensory area or merely a small area over the first dorsal interosseous (R_1).

Of greater functional value to the patient is the ability to localize a site of sensation with the eyes closed. The blindfolded patient is asked to identify the exact area touched by the examiner.

Testing can be with a pin prick or scratch (pain) or cotton (light touch). Testing should begin at the tips of the palmar surface of the fingers where sensation is most acute. Quantitative testing has been advocated in which numerous fibers of different stiffness (e.g., horsehair or nylon) are pressed perpendicular to the skin until they bend. The patient, with his eyes closed, identifies the point of pressure and specifically records the exact site.

Two-point discrimination (Weber test) involves touching the skin with two blunt points simultaneously, with the two points placed along a longitudinal line of the finger. The patient, with his eyes closed, immediately specifies whether he feels one or two points. The number is varied according to the separation. If two times out of three the patient does not recognize one or two points correctly, proprioceptive impairment is implied. This two-point discrimination instrument can be made by spreading a paper clip. The normal distances on the palmar surfaces of the fingers that can be discerned consist of the index finger, 2 to 4 mm.; the little finger, 3 to 5 mm.; the dorsum of the hand, 6 to 12 mm.

A failure above 10 mm. implies a loss of sufficient significance to impair precision hand grip. This test requires judgment on the part of the patient and therefore demands intelligence, cooperation, and patience and does not primarily test nerve sensation.

Sympathetic innervation is also specific. Only an injury to a nerve proximal to the entry of the sympathetic nerve into the peripheral nerve will fail to damage the sudomotor function of that nerve (Fig. 59). The denervated portion of the hand fails to perspire, and the skin feels dry. The specific loss of perspiration can be photographed by painting the hand with an alcohol solution of cobalt chloride, then causing the patient to perspire.

Immediately after denervation the hand is warm, presumably due to paresis of the vasomotor nerves. The hand gets cold after three to four weeks.

Tactile sensory loss can best be determined by testing hand function. Recognizing numerous small objects such as screws, pin, tacks, or paper

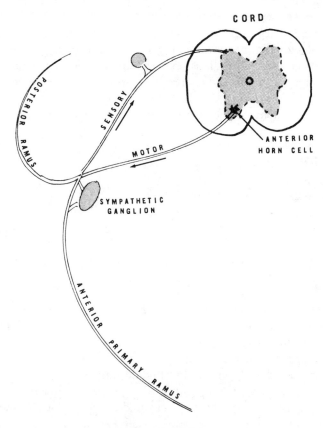

FIGURE 59. Formation of peripheral nerve. A peripheral nerve is mixed with the anterior motor and dorsal sensory fibers united. The sympathetic fibers join distal to their union and any interruption distal to the sympathetic entry will cause sudomotor loss.

clips or the texture or size of objects and observing the patient's ability to manipulate these objects during the test are practical tests of sensory function. Comparison with the normal hand and setting a time factor for each test makes them quantitative.

Voluntary muscle testing is done manually. Some form of quantitative grading must be established—from total paralysis to contraction against resistance to normal. Testing isolated muscle function may be difficult. It is better to test hand function such as finger flexion, thumb adduction to the index, opposition of thumb to little finger, and spreading the fingers.

The three major motor nerves are thus tested:
1. Median—flexor carpi radialis, flexor digitorum profundus of the index, flexor pollicis longus, flexor digitorum superficialis, and abductor pollicis brevis.
2. Ulnar—flexor carpi ulnaris, flexor digitorum profundus of the little finger, abductor digiti quinti, adductor pollicis, first dorsal interosseous.
3. Radial—extensor carpi radialis, extensor digitorum communis, extensor pollicis longus, extensor indicis proprius, triceps, and brachioradialis.

In summary, lesions of the three nerves of the hand result in the following:

Severance of the *radial* nerve:
1. Wrist drop.
2. Inability to extend proximal phalanges.
3. Inability to extend or abduct the thumb.
4. Hypesthesia of the dorsum of the hand (see Fig. 58). May have no sensory loss.
5. Absence of brachioradialis reflex (and possibly triceps reflex).

Severance of *median* nerve:
1. Hypesthesia of the palmar area (see Fig. 58). (Anesthesia is usually complete only on the palmar and dorsal aspect of terminal phalanges of the index and middle fingers.)
2. Weakness of wrist flexors and pronation.
3. Inability to flex thumb, index, and middle fingers.
4. Difficulty in opposing tip of thumb to tip of other fingers.
5. Slight hyperextension of the first and middle fingers at the metacarpophalangeal joint due to unopposed finger extensors.
6. Functional loss of precision grip, difficulty picking up small objects, inability to identify small objects when blind-folded, weakened power grip due to failure of thumb stabilization action.

Severance of the *ulnar* nerve:

1. Hypesthesia of ulnar aspect of hand (see Fig. 58).
2. Inability to flex distal phalanges of fourth and fifth fingers.
3. Loss of ulnar wrist flexion.
4. Inability to hold paper between thumb and index finger.
5. Weakness in finger spreading.
6. Difficulty forming perfect letter *O* with thumb and index finger.
7. Ring and little fingers hyperextend (30 degrees) at metacarpophalangeal joints.
8. Functional loss of writing due to loss of sensation of little finger, poor pinch grip, and loss of power grip due to inability to wrap fingers around an object. There is loss of thumb adductor.

Damage to the median nerve presents the greatest impairment as it supplies the sensation to the major portion of the palm and first three fingers and the motor function of power grip between the thumb, index, and middle fingers. Ulnar nerve damage causes a serious impairment to the person who performs finely coordinated activities such as playing the piano and typing. Damage to both the ulnar and median nerves gravely impairs total hand function and is frequently seen following lacerations at the wrist.

The anatomy of a mixed peripheral nerve is shown in Figure 60. A mixed peripheral nerve contains fibers of different sizes having both sensory and motor functions. Fifty percent of a nerve is axon and the rest is connective tissue. The blood supply enters the nerve and branches longitudinally in both directions within the sheath. Pathology of the injured nerve depends upon the type and extent of the injury. Contusion or stretching causes swelling and hemorrhage *within* the nerve with possible residual external and internal scar formation. Laceration, whether complete or partial, causes a scar *within* the nerve that spreads longitudinally in both directions from the cut portion. The extent of the scar cannot be ascertained at the time of the injury. With complete nerve disruption, axon degeneration proceeds distally to its myoneural junction. This is known as wallerian degeneration. Some retrograde degeneration also occurs in the next one or two nodes of Ranvier.

Five degrees of nerve damage have been documented by Sunderland. First degree injury constitutes loss of conductivity of the axon *without* loss in continuity. This can result from momentary violence, prolonged compression, or petechial hemorrhage in or near the sheath. There is usually loss of motor function and tone with reduction of proprioception, but touch and pain sensation remain. Touch is affected more than pain sensation so there is more anesthesia than analgesia. Recovery may occur within several days and is usually complete within three months.

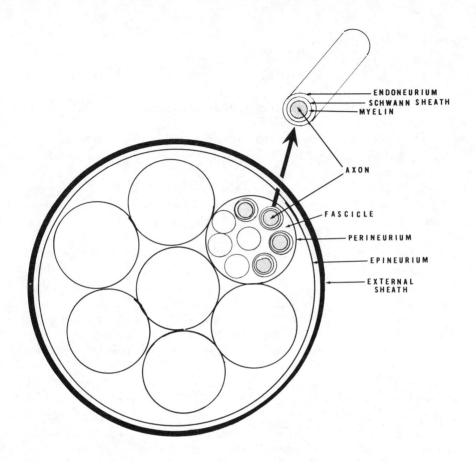

FIGURE 60. Peripheral nerve (schematic). In cross section a nerve is composed of many axons grouped into a fascicle. Each axon is surrounded by myelin enclosed within a sheath of Schwann. This is in turn coated with endoneurium which is composed of longitudinal collagen strips. Perineurium binds the fascicles which are in turn bound together by epineurium. The entire nerve is covered by an external sheath.

In second degree injury, axons are severed. Wallerian degeneration occurs but the endoneural tubes remain intact permitting axon regeneration within their own tubules. The effect is complete motor, sensory, and sympathetic loss within 20 hours at which point there is *no* more reaction to electrical stimulation. Muscular atrophy is usual. *Chromatolysis* occurs with central degeneration of the anterior horn cell and the posterior root of the sensory nerves. Since the root is more involved than the anterior horn cell, there is greater sensory loss and slower sensory recovery than motor loss or recovery. Because the tubule remains intact, no suture is necessary and recovery is usually complete.

Third degree injuries disorganize the internal structure of the funiculus and interrupt both the axon and the tubule. The epineurium and perineurium may remain intact. Due to hemorrhage within the funiculus

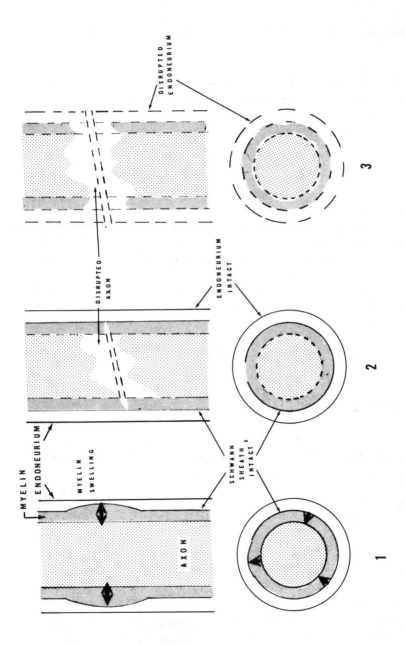

FIGURE 61. Degrees of nerve injury. (1) A loss of conductivity *without* break in continuity. There is swelling of the myelin within an intact Schwann sheath that compresses the axon (arrows). (2) The axon is severed but the endoneural sheath (tubule) remains intact. Schwann sheath may also remain intact. Regeneration of the axon is within its own tubule. (3) The entire fascicle is disrupted—the axon, Schwann sheath, and endoneurium. Regeneration frequently meets obstruction due to fibrosis occurring at the severed ends. (4) and (5) All the funiculi within the fascicles (the entire nerve) are disrupted including the perineurium and epineurium.

and endoneural damage, ultimate *fibrosis* can be predicted. Recovery depends upon the obstruction met by the regenerating axon. The residual loss depends upon the site of damage—the more distal the site, the less the loss.

Fourth through fifth degree disruption of *all* the funiculi of the nerve trunk causes total loss of motor, sensory, and sympathetic function. Microscopically, differentiation of epineurium from perineurium is not possible. The nerve is *divided* and formation of a neuroma is common. Even good surgical approximation under optimal conditions results in limited functional recovery.

The degrees of disruption have been termed: (a) axonapraxia—physiological interruption with intact nerve and no wallerian degeneration; (b) axonotmesis—axon disruption with degeneration but intact sheaths; and (c) neurotmesis—disruption of both axon and sheath.

During degeneration a reaction occurs within the anterior horn cell (Fig. 61) which forms *axoplasm.* This substance stimulates regrowth distally from the proximal segment and usually begins in two to three weeks. This explains the electromyographic findings in which degeneration fibrillation occurs three weeks after injury followed later by polyphasic waves which indicate regeneration. The type and extent of nerve disruption cannot be accurately established clinically. An injury originally considered to be a physiological interruption without discontinuity but which does not heal within four to six weeks should be explored surgically. By this time a physiological disruption usually shows signs of healing. Complete disruption now is evident by electromyogram. Complete nerve disruption ultimately results in muscular atrophy, fibrosis, and skin and joint changes.

Following nerve interruption, changes occur in the muscle. After six weeks the fibers begin kinking and the striations fade. After three months there is an increase in connective tissue which totally replaces muscle by fibrous tissue in approximately two years. Wasting is noted about four to six weeks after the nerve lesion, spreads rapidly after two months, and is maximal after three months. Deep tendon reflexes diminish as atrophy progresses.

Treatment

Although it is not the intent to discuss the techniques of surgery, types of suture material, nor the choice of instruments in this monograph, there are concepts of care for injuries that must be followed by any physician caring for the patient during an emergency situation. Adherence to these concepts by the doctor helps the patient to reach the hand surgeon with a better possibility for functional recovery.

Primary suture of a divided nerve is to be discouraged and must be done *only* in the most ideal situation. A primary suture does *not* necessarily give better sensory recovery than does secondary suture done four to eight weeks after wound healing. Initially it is impossible to determine the extent of *internal* scarring expected proximally and distally to the lesion. The severed ends are usually irregular (jagged) and the epineurium too friable to permit good sutured opposition of the severed ends.

Primary suture should be considered only when:

1. There is a clean cut with minimal tissue damage.
2. Both nerve ends are easily located.
3. Wound edges can be easily approximated and sutured *without* tension.
4. There is no infection.
5. All proper suture material and instruments are present.
6. A competent experienced surgeon is available.

Initial surgery of the severed nerve is for identification, close approximation, and placement of a localizing suture for later recovery and identification.

Proper initial care of the injured hand should ultimately insure recovery of maximum function. The initial treatment frequently determines the ultimate recovery, even though the final definitive treatment is of the highest quality.

Skin closure or coverage by suture or graft is the basis of the primary care of the injured hand. This prevents infection and protects the exposed deep tissues. Closure obviously implies careful cleaning and debridement. *Care of the nerve supply takes precedence over all the deep tissues.* Surgical reconstruction or definitive repair is carried out as soon as local tissue conditions permit.

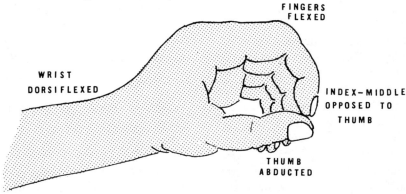

FINGERS
FLEXED

WRIST
DORSIFLEXED

INDEX–MIDDLE
OPPOSED TO
THUMB

THUMB
ABDUCTED

FIGURE 62. Functional position of the hand. This position should be sought during immobilization of the hand by splinting or bandaging. Deviation from this position is obviously permitted for specific medical reasons.

During the period of paralysis following nerve injury and during recovery of the hand following surgical repair, certain principles must be followed. The hand must be elevated constantly to prevent edema. All unaffected muscles and joints must be moved actively through their range of motion. Warm soaks may be applied locally, and the hand and fingers must be splinted in a physiological position when not moving (Fig. 62). Materials for splinting are numerous and easily adapted.

Recovery in children is more favorable than in adults and complete recovery is possible even after a period of five years. Recovery of high quality sensation in the sutured nerve, however, is rare.

NERVE COMPRESSION

Compression of a nerve may cause local injury and inflammation with resultant symptoms and disability. Compression may be caused by an anatomical encroachment upon the normal course of the nerve. The intensity and duration of the compression will determine the amount of swelling within the sheath or damage to and degeneration of the axon and its tubule, with resultant fibrosis.

Compression neuropathy, entrapment, usually causes pain described as sharp or burning and is associated with hyperesthesia, hypesthesia, or paresthesia. Nerve tenderness is usual. Characteristically this pain occurs during rest and at night.

Median Nerve Compression

The median nerve can be entrapped at numerous sites in its normal route down the arm from the cervical roots to its terminus. The most common site of compression is at the wrist under the transverse carpal ligament where it accompanies the flexor tendons of the fingers (see Figs. 12, 13, and 14). This is why primary suture may be difficult as the palmaris longus may be sutured to the nerve in error.

At this site the nerve supplies motor fibers to the muscles of the thumb (opponens pollicis and abductor pollicis brevis and the first and second lumbrical muscles) and sensation to the midpalm and the palmar area of the first three and a half digits (see Fig. 58) as well as the sensation of the dorsal tips of these fingers. Variations exist in which the entire hand is supplied by the median nerve or much of the hand normally supplied by the median nerve is supplied by the ulnar.

Median nerve compression at the wrist causes motor weakness of the:

1. Abductor pollici brevis—elevation of the thumb at right angle to the plane of the palm. Clinical evaluation is unreliable as this movement

can be mimicked by combined action of the flexor pollicis brevis (ulnar nerve) and the abductor pollicis longus (radial nerve).

2. Opponens pollicis, which approximates tip to thumb to tip of little finger. This opposition can be mimicked by flexor pollicis brevis and the adductor pollicis (both innervated by the ulnar nerve).
3. First and second lumbrical muscles, which extend the fingers at the interphalangeal joint with metacarpophalangeal joint hyperextended. This action can be substituted by the extensor communis digitorum when the metacarpophalangeal joint hyperextension is eliminated.
4. Flexor pollicis brevis, which has a dual innervation—median and ulnar—and thus no evaluation import.

Compression of the median nerve at the transverse carpal ligament causes numbness, burning, and ultimately tingling of the first three fingers. Symptoms are most common in women and are usually unilateral but both hands may be affected. Symptoms usually occur during the night or early hours of the morning and awaken the patient. Relief is sought by shaking, elevating, or immersing the hands in hot water. Pain may ascend the arm causing the examiner to suspect a cervical dorsal outlet syndrome or cervical radiculitis.

Diminished sensation may result in clumsiness which may be accompanied by weakness and "dropping things." Cyanosis is noted frequently. Initially absence of objective findings frequently suggests a diagnosis of hysteria or neurosis. Subjective complaints without physical findings may be the forerunner of multiple sclerosis but also should alert one to the possibility of radiculitis from cervical diskogenic disease, neurovascular compression of the cervical dorsal outlet syndrome, or other peripheral neuropathies.

The initial objective findings consist of impaired sensation of a pin prick over the median nerve distribution area—usually the index and middle fingers with the thumb less frequently involved. Loss of temperature, light touch, and position sense is uncommon. Slight weakness without atrophy is difficult to evaluate. Atrophy is usually noted first in the thenar eminence in the short abductor of the thumb when the condition is more severe or prolonged.

The diagnosis of *carpal tunnel syndrome* is made by (1) the typical history of nocturnal paresthesias and the characteristic painful numbness and tingling; (2) objective sensory and motor loss on examination; (3) reproduction of the symptoms by sustained wrist flexion or extension or by manual compression of the radial and ulnar arteries; (4) relief of symptoms by immobilizing the wrist in a neutral position; and (5) prolongation of nerve conduction velocity on electomyographic studies. It is not desirable to await objective sensory and motor deficit before instituting treatment.

The characteristic noctural paresthesias relieved by wearing a daytime splint on the wrist defies explanation. Reproduction of the symptoms by maintaining wrist flexion is paradoxical if pressure upon the nerve is implicated because pressure within the carpal tunnel is three times greater with the wrist extended than flexed (Fig. 63).

Inflating a sphygmomanometer cuff around the arm or manually compressing the radial and ulnar artery at the wrist causes an unpleasant tingling and numbness in the fingers. Release of the pressure results in a "pins and needles" sensation lasting as long as five to ten seconds. Pressure upon the median nerve at the wrist causes no dysesthesia; therefore the mechanism must be considered to be vascular.

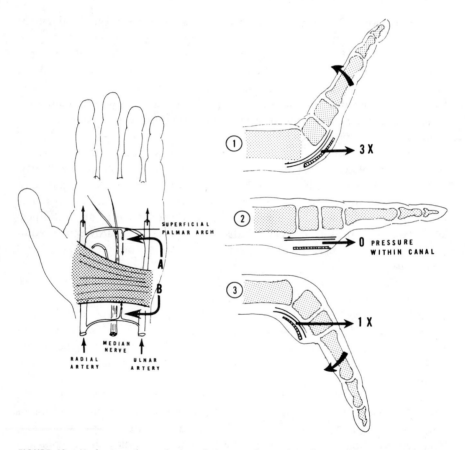

FIGURE 63. Mechanism of parethesiae of the carpal tunnel syndrome. The large figure shows the arterial circulation of the median nerve receiving a small branch distally from the superficial palmar arch (A) and a branch proximally from the ulnar artery (B). Compression can occur distally from occupational pressures on the palm and proximally from prolonged flexion or extension of the wrist with simultaneous finger flexion compressing the small proximal arterial branch. (1) Wrist extension (dorsiflexion) which creates three times the pressure within the carpal tunnel as is found during wrist flexion (3). During relaxation (2) there is release of the arterial compression.

It can be postulated that the nerve becomes ischemic during the day from repeated wrist dorsiflexion with simultaneous contraction of the finger flexors. This constricts the tunnel space during the day with vascular release during rest at night when the paresthesias appear. Preventing wrist motion during the day by splinting prevents compression and thus does not cause ischemia. No release phenomenon occurs at night. Space-occupying lesions, such as a Colles' fracture, Smith fracture, dislocated carpal bone, tumor, rheumatoid arthritis, and tenosynovitis of finger flexors, can compromise the tunnel space and cause nerve entrapment. Treatment requires that these be eliminated when possible.

It must always be kept in mind that the "usual" median nerve sensory distribution and motor innervation to four and a half of the muscles of the hand (*opponens pollicis, abductor pollicis brevis, first and second lumbrical muscles, and the superficial head of the flexor pollicis brevis*) may vary tremendously. An "all median nerve hand" is frequent wherein the entire hand is supplied by the median nerve with no ulnar innervation. An "all ulnar hand" also occurs. Only accurate diagnosis by electromyogram with percutaneous electrical stimulation can clarify these variants.

Treatment. The basis for treatment is suggested by the postulated mechanism. If no space-occupying lesions, such as a Colles' or Smith fracture or dislocated carpal bone, are discernible, it must be assumed there is a mechanical etiology of daytime activities requiring prolonged wrist dorsiflexion with simultaneous gripping.

Conservative treatment requires the wrist to be splinted in a neutral position throughout the day and, preferably also, the night. Merely splinting at night does *not* relieve the symptoms. If the patient's daytime activities are strenuous and cannot be minimized and a splint cannot be continually worn, conservative treatment will be ineffective. Under these circumstances, early surgery may be desirable. Motor impairment indicates the need for early surgery as sensory return is usual after surgical decompression, but motor return is variable and usually incomplete.

The *entire* width of the transverse carpal ligament must be surgically divided. Failure most commonly occurs when there is incomplete section of the ligament due to the surgeon's unawareness of the width of the ligament. Exposure must be extensive, but the skin incision must be as small as possible to minimize scarring. Keloid formation is common in this area. During surgery if the synovium of the finger flexors is found to be "boggy" or thickened, it should be removed.

If a patient has an occupation that requires handling tools in the palm of the hand with constant gripping and pressure, a protective pad should be worn. Injection of steroids under the carpal ligament has some diagnostic value but limited therapeutic value. Ultrasound treatment has proven disappointing. Use of oral anti-inflammatory drugs and diuretics during splinting is beneficial.

Median Nerve Compression: Pronator Teres Syndrome

The median nerve can be compressed in its passage below the elbow as it passes through the two heads of the pronator teres muscle before it goes under the proximal edge of the flexor digitorum muscle. The usual cause of compression is direct trauma such as a direct blow or carrying a heavy object on the upper forearm. The mechanism is postulated to be a "kinking" of the nerve against the sharp edge of the sublimis muscle (Fig. 64) with the nerve being lifted and thus angulated by the ulnar half of the pronator teres.

In the forearm the median nerve supplies the pronator teres, flexor carpi radialis, palmaris longus, and the digitorum superficialis. Just distal to the pronator muscle, the median nerve sends branches to the ulnar half of the flexor digitorum profundus, the flexor pollicis longus, and the pronator quadratus.

The muscles supplied by the median nerve along its course in the forearm can be tested clinically to determine impaired function, but confusion is possible.

The pronator teres pronates the forearm with the elbow prevented from rotation. The muscle can be palpated below the antecubital space. Substitution can be performed by the brachioradialis and long flexors of the forearm. The palmaris longus and flexor carpi radialis flex the wrist with the tendons palpable (see Fig. 15). The palmaris longus may substitute for the flexor carpi radialis.

Flexor digitorum sublimis flexes the proximal interphalangeal joints with the wrist and the metacarpophalangeal joints immobilized in a neutral position. Motion can be tested but tendons are not palpable. Flexor digitorum profundus of the index and third finger (the fourth and fifth flexors are innervated by the ulnar nerve) flexes the distal phalanx with the wrist and proximal phalanx immobilized. This motion can be tested but the tendons cannot be palpated. The ulnar nerve may innervate the long (third) finger, thus the index finger is the most reliable to test. Tenodesis action by the flexor tendons can substitute both sublimis and profundus action during wrist extension, so the wrist must be immobilized in a neutral position when testing.

Flexor pollicis longus flexes the distal phalanx of the thumb. Extension of the wrist and the first metacarpal can, by tenodesis action, produce mechanical thumb flexion. The pronator quadratus is not testable.

Compression of the median nerve at this level will simulate the carpal tunnel syndrome. The patient will complain of burning and pain of

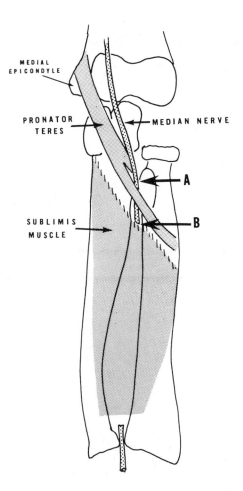

FIGURE 64. Median nerve compression, pronator teres. The median nerve passes between the heads of the pronator teres then passes under the edge of the flexor digitorum sublimis muscle. Pressure at (A) may occur due to repetitive pronation with simultaneous forceful finger flexion. The nerve can be elevated under the fibrous edge of the sublimis muscle (B). Direct pressure may be exerted at the antecubital area.

the first three digits, possible weakness of the thumb opposition and first three finger flexors, and aggravation of the pain when pronation of the forearm with a tightly clenched fist is resisted.

Differentiation of compression at the transverse carpal ligament from compression at the forearm is suggested by the latter having sensory impairment at the thenar eminence, whereas entrapment at the wrist causes sensory impairment of the flexor surface of the thumb and the first two and a half digits. Pronation of the forearm aggravates the symptoms and there is deep tenderness of the forearm. After prolonged compression, weakness of wrist pronation may be elicited.

Treatment requires rest by splinting to prevent pronation. Relief is possible by injecting the site of tenderness with steroids and procaine. When the condition fails to respond to conservative treatment or if an impending Volkmann's contracture is the cause, surgical decompression with or without neurolysis may be necessary.

Ulnar Nerve Compression

The ulnar nerve is subjected to compression at numerous sites along its course. At the wrist the ulnar nerve enters the hand in a shallow trough between the pisiform bone and the hook of the hamate bone. The floor is a thin layer of ligament and muscle, and its roof is the volar carpal ligament and palmaris longus muscle (Fig. 65). Upon distal emergence through the tunnel is gives off two cutaneous branches that supply sensation of the ulnar side of the palm, the fouth and fifth fingers (see Fig. 58). The deep branch innervates the muscles of the hypothenar eminence, the third and fourth lumbricals, all the interossei, the adductor pollicis, and the deep head of the flexor pollicis brevis.

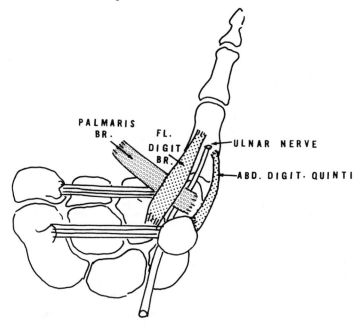

FIGURE 65. Ulnar nerve entry into hand at wrist (Guyon's canal).

Three lesions can occur at the wrist: (1) trunk, which is both motor and sensory; (2) superficial, which causes predominantly sensor impairment; and (3) deep, which causes only motor impairment. Usually, deep and trunk lesions occur simultaneously.

Etiology is usually trauma, which may be a single acute episode or a repetitive trauma such as operating a pneumatic drill. A Colles' or Smith fracture may cause entrapment symptoms. Also gout or benign swelling such as a ganglion have been implicated.

Symptoms will depend on the site of nerve entrapment. Trunk involvement will cause a "burning" sensation in the sensory area of the fourth and fifth fingers. The sensation may vary from an "uncomfortable numbness" to severe "burning." Motor weakness may be described as "clumsiness" in performing fine movements. "Pinch" strength of the thumb is noted and atrophy of the interossei may become apparent with deepening of the interosseous grooves in the dorsum of the hand. Some thenar muscle atrophy may be noted. In deep branch involvement pain is possible but rare. Symptoms are essentially those of weakness, especially in testing abduction and adduction of the fingers, flexion of the metacarpophalangeal joints, and adduction of the thumb. Motor weakness of the little finger is apparent.

Treatment may merely require steroid and analgesic infiltration by injection into the cubital tunnel, which is both diagnostic and therapeutic. When time and conservative treatment fails to alter progressive weakness, surgical decompression must be considered. The ulnar nerve may be injured or entrapped at the elbow in the cubital tunnel. If the symptoms are a result of late sequelae of an injury it is sometimes termed a "tardy ulnar palsy." Since the ulnar nerve is formed by the lower trunk of the brachial plexus (C_7 and T_1), lesions above the elbow and at the wrist must always be considered when ulnar nerve symptoms are present.

The nerve passes through a groove behind the medial epicondyle, covered by a fibrous sheath that forms the "cubital tunnel," and then enters the forearm between the two heads of the flexor carpi ulnaris. In its passage down the forearm it supplies the flexor carpi ulnaris and the flexor digitorum profundus. The wrist and hand innervations are as noted in the previous section of the ulnar nerve. Because the ulnar nerve is relatively exposed in a groove where it lies on a bony surface covered merely by thin fascia and skin, it is exposed to trauma. The floor of the tunnel is formed by the medial ligament and the medial tip of the trochlea. The roof is the arcuate ligament which is taut at $90°$ of elbow flexion and slack in elbow extension. The medial ligament bulges in flexion, and thus the ulnar nerve undergoes "physiological" compression during elbow flexion. Prolonged periods of extreme elbow flexion should thus be avoided.

With the arm abducted (as in an arm board for intravenous injections), full supination of the forearm pulls the tunnel away from pressure (Fig. 66). Pronation encourages compression. In extreme elbow flexion and external pressure damage is more probable. As depicted in Figure 66, the sensory fibers of the ulnar nerve are more superficial than its motor fibers, and thus sensory symptoms are earlier and more predominant. Damage to

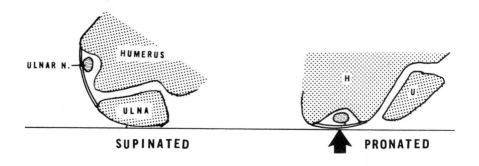

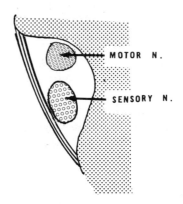

FIGURE 66. Cubital tunnel—ulnar nerve. In the supinated elbow the ulnar nerve is removed from possible compression, whereas pronation encourages pressure. The lower figure depicts the sensory component of the nerve as compared with the motor fibers.

the ulnar nerve is more probable in the case of alcoholism, diabetes, vitamin deficiencies, or malignancy.

Trauma may be acute pressure or repeated minor pressures produced, for example, by leaning on a hard surface or by "tethering" of the nerve during forceful elbow flexion when there is a malalignment of the forearm to the humerus. Occasionally the cubital fossa is shallow or the fascial covering is deficient, and the ulnar nerve "slips out."

Compression can be classified as (1) acute, resulting from a single episode of force, (2) subacute, resulting from external pressure over a limited period, or (3) chronic, resulting from pressure from lesions within the canal, such as osteoarthritic changes, rheumatoid arthritis, ganglion, and soft tissue tumors.

The degree of palsy (McGowen) is listed as: Grade I, paresthesiae and minor hypoesthesia; Grade II, weakness and wasting of interossei with incomplete hypoesthesia; and Grade III, paralysis of interossei and medial two lumbricals and severe wasting of the hypothenar and adductor pollicis ("clawing" of the ring and little finger).

The patient most frequently complains of "burning" pain in the fourth and fifth fingers. Hyperaesthesia may ultimately be replaced by numbness and weakness initially termed "clumsiness." Radiation of this pain from the elbow entrapment has been claimed to interscapular area but the mechanism for this is not clear.

Weakness is noted in the intrinsic muscles causing hyperextension of the metacarpophalangeal joints, weakness of separation (abduction) of the fingers, and weakness of flexor carpi ulnaris and flexor digitorum profundus to the fourth and fifth fingers. Atrophy may ultimately be noted in the hypothenar eminence. The presence of weakness of the flexor carpi ulnaris and flexor digitorum profundus of the fourth and fifth fingers places the lesion above (proximal to) the wrist. Electromyography can clarify this location.

Treatment of a conservative nature such as pressure pads over the fossa, avoidance of pressure in writing postures, and avoidance of excessive flexion has frequently been discredited in favor of early surgical transplantation. However, Payan in 1970 did electrophysiological studies that confirmed sensory recovery to be as rapid and complete following conservative treatment as surgical transposition.

Lesions more proximal, at the cervical spine and supraclavicular area (the medial cord), are reproducible by cervical motions and thoracic outlet maneuvers.

The deformity noted in a complete ulnar nerve palsy is (1) flexion deformity of the fourth and fifth fingers due to lumbrical palsy, (2) interosseous atrophy, (3) flattening of the hypothenar eminence, and (4) concavity of web between the thumb and index fingers due to atrophy of the first dorsal interosseous and the adductor pollicis.

The flexor carpi ulnaris can be tested by flexing the wrist in an ulnar direction and palpating the tendon at the wrist. More simply it can be tested by resisting *ab*duction of the fifth finger during which the flexor carpi ulnaris synergistically fixes the wrist so that its tendon can be palpated. This action occurs even with paralysis of the abductor minimi digiti.

Checking flexor digitorum profundus function is best done at the fifth finger and involves flexion of the distal phalanx since the fourth flexor digitorum profundus is frequently innervated by the median nerve.

Tests for the oponens digiti minimi (bringing fifth finger across palmar aspect of ring finger), palmar interossei (adducting fingers against resistance), adductor pollicis (adductor sweep test—sweeping thumb across metacarpal heads), and Froment's sign (grasping a piece of paper between thumb and radial side of palm) are not clinically satisfactory. Individual function by direct palpation and visible contraction make it difficult to discern substitution.

The test for the first dorsal interosseous (ulnar nerve C_8 and T_1) is clear and easily performed by abducting the index finger. Care, however, must be exercised that the abduction motion is not performed by the extensor indicis proprius. When the fingers are in a slight degree of flexion, abduction can be done by the flexor digitorum profundus. To competently examine the first dorsal interosseous, proper position and motion of the finger must be assured.

Traction Nerve Injuries

Traction nerve injuries notoriously have a poor prognosis. A test is possible to distinguish preganglionic from postganglionic lesions by electromyogram sensory conduction time determination. In a totally anesthetic hand, the ability to elicit a sensory action potential on distal electrical stimulation indicates an intact pathway to the sensory ganglion. Absence of action potential implies that the lesion is postganglionic and has a better prognosis. A preganglionic lesion offers a hopeless prognosis and indicates that immediate repair should be undertaken to restore function rather than waiting for nerve recovery. In brachial plexus traction injuries, upper root lesions have a better prognosis than lower plexus and the patient should show signs of recovery within one year.

Causalgia

This term is now established as a specific disease entity but it still escapes definition, causation, and singular terminology. The term is derived from *kausos* (heat) and *algo* (pain), as it is a painful state frequently described by the patient as a burning sensation.

The numerous terms now closely associated with the causalgic syndrome were initially described by Weir Mitchell in 1872 who described the burning pain in the sensory distribution of a nerve near a penetrating missile wound. The intensity of the pain which varied from "trivial" to "excruciating and unbearable" resulted in the classification of *minor* or *major* causalgia.

Homans in 1940 initiated the term *minor* as a vascular mechanism in which he felt the pain was related to both vasomotor and sudomotor autonomic hyperactivity with resultant osteoporosis, reflex dystrophy, and Sudeck's atrophy. Volkmann in 1882 described a painful post-traumatic rarefaction of a bone. Destot in 1898 observed pain in a foot and ankle several months after a severe sprain in which osteoporosis was visible on x-ray. Sudeck in 1900 described the same condition but added other signs such as edema, coldness, and cyanosis to the presence of pain.

Causalgic pain is constant, deep, diffuse, and intense; characteristically described as burning. Women are more often affected than men. The pain is intensified by exposure to cold, heat, moving air currents, or light touching. In the hand, it is most prevalent in the median nerve distribution. The patient prohibits any passive motion of the part and avoids any active movement. The facies of the patient depicts the subjective severity of the pain and the affected part often is kept wrapped in moist loose dressing, compresses are applied, the part is held elevated and is kept away from all contact.

The pain may immediately follow an injury such as cortex fracture, sprain, penetrating wound, or minor nerve injury. Not infrequently, a delay of weeks may follow a minor injury before severe subjective pain is alleged by the patient. Severe pain may even be claimed in the absence of any objective findings.

The extremity involved may show vasospasm or vasodilatation with dilatation noted first. The hand is pink, warm, and dry. The condition may then progress to vasospasm (constriction) with the hand becoming cold, bluish, and moist. Progression ultimately causes the skin to become glossy (shiny), the intrinsic muscle to undergo atrophy, and the joints to stiffen. Fortunately, most cases of causalgia terminate or are aborted therapeutically before the final stages are reached.

The mechanism of causalgia remains obscure. The sympathetic system is obviously involved. *Pain is the primary causative factor* with all other tissue changes secondary. The susceptible patient usually has a low pain threshold and emotional lability. An injury causes infiltration of exudate into the tissues which cannot be removed since the patient avoids any movement. *Inactivity* (immobility) becomes the secondary major causative factor. Further venous congestion and lymphatic stasis results in ultimate organization of the protein rich exudate. Fibrosis, chronic edema, and osteoporosis result. The cycle is self-perpetuating so long as the pain which causes inactivity persists.

The causes of causalgia are as numerous as the varieties of this syndrome. The syndrome is termed Sudeck's atrophy, causalgia(minor or major), post-traumatic osteoporosis, myocardial infarction, painful shoulder, swollen atrophic hand associated with cervical radiculitis, hand-shoulder syndrome of hemiplegia, and so forth. The syndrome portrays varying degrees of reflex physiological reaction, both vasomotor and sudomotor, to an inciting internal or external noxious agent.

Treatment is essentially the interruption of the causative cycle and must be initiated early and energetically. Although it is estimated that approximately 60 percent of all patients make a spontaneous recovery, the rapidity and completeness of recovery is influenced by the efficacy of the treatment.

Prevention is the treatment of choice. In any injury to an extremity, immobilization must be exact and comfortable with the proximal and distal joints left free and their movements encouraged. The part must be elevated to prevent venous congestion and dependent edema. Pain must be controlled by appropriate medication. Aspirin has analgesic as well as other benefits not fully understood and must be administered in large and periodic doses, taken on a full stomach, and used with antacid medicine to prevent gastric irritation. A stronger analgesic may be necessary. Trigger areas when found can be infiltrated with a local anesthetic or sprayed with ethyl chloride. A painful scar or neuroma may need surgical removal but if surgery is once attempted unsuccessfully, it *must not be repeated.*

Perineural infusion of the "trigger area" has recently been advocated. The localized area is surgically prepped, and a large bore needle is inserted into the area until the symptoms are reproduced. Then a flexible vena catheter is inserted through the needle, 0.5 ml of 0.5 percent lidocaine is infiltrated. If the symptoms are relieved, the needle is removed leaving the vena catheter inserted and repeated injections of lidocaine every 3 to 4 hours for 2 to 3 weeks are administered.

Selective large-nerve electrical stimulation proximal to the lesion is applied. A 0.1 millisecond unidirectional square wave (100 Hertz voltage) is applied for 2 to 3 minutes giving relief for 2 to 12 hours, during which time active physical therapy can be administered.

Recently there have been encouraging reports of marked benefit in the treatment of causalgia by using chlorpromazine (Thorazine) orally or by intramuscular route. Dosage varies from 50 to 400 mg daily followed by maintenance doses of 25 mg b.i.d. During early administration of chlorpromazine, hospitalization is recommended because of secondary blood pressure changes that can occur; however, complications from chlorpromazine are controllable and not serious.

Insofar as sympathetic discharges are thought to originate in the midbrain a "short circuiting" into the sensory nerve of the peripheral nerves is thought to be a sequence of the etiological injury. Chlorpromazine is considered to act at the central level.

To minimize venous congestion and stasis edema, isometric muscular contraction should be started immediately. This type of exercise does not move the involved joints nor elongate the inflamed tissues, but does cause the muscles to enhance venous return and mobilize the lymphatic circulation, thus removing the edema. Uninvolved joints must be actively moved through the full range of motion frequently during waking hours.

When unbearable pain prevents the patient's cooperation, the cervicothoracic sympathetic innervation must be interrupted. This can be done by blocking the stellate ganglion with Novocain or one of its derivatives. On rare occasions where a chemical block is effective but its benefit of short duration, a surgical interruption of the sympathetic nerves is indicated. This intervention is rarely required. Even successful interruption of the sympathetic innervation does not permit the neglect of active motion, elevation, pain medication, and tranquilizers. *Cure cannot be achieved without patient cooperation.*

The presence of secondary gains when the alleged injury is industrial or a compensable personal injury adds a different factor. Pathological malingering has not medically been clarified as either conscious or unconscious, but the end result is that the patient has a residual disability and has expended large financial sums. Treatment is identical medically but, to be effective, the motivation of secondary gains by maintaining the disability must be removed.

Nerve Root Involvement

Weakness and numbness of the fingers present differential diagnostic problems between root irritation from cervical degenerative arthrosis and carpal tunnel median nerve compression. Diagnosis is especially difficult

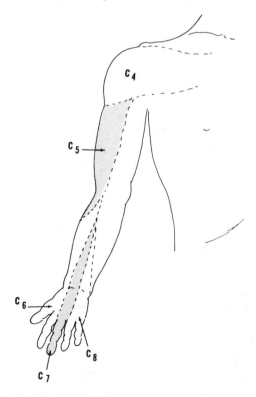

FIGURE 67. Cervical root sensory map. Depicts the usual sensory areas supplied by cervical roots C_4 through C_8.

when there is atrophy and weakness of the thenar prominence *and* x-ray evidence of disk degeneration between C_5, C_6, and C_7.

Attributing the symptoms to cervical root irritation is refuted by the following. The C_6 root which emerges between C_5 and C_6 does *not* innervate the muscles of the hand or fingers. It motorvates the wrist (in conjunction with C_7) through the pronator teres, extensor carpi radialis longus and brevis, flexor carpi radialis and ulnaris. Thus, involvement of the C_6 root alone may cause hypesthesia of the thumb and index fingers (Fig. 67) and weakness of the wrist flexor and wrist radial extensor but *no* atrophy of weakness of the fingers. C_7 root involvement weakens the finger extensors and long thumb abductor (the latter receives branches from C_8).

The finger flexors are primarily innervated by C_8 and T_1 with some branches from C_7. The opponens pollicis, abductor pollicis brevis, flexor pollicis brevis, and the intrinsic muscles are essentially innervated by C_8 and T_1. Thus, when there is numbness of the thumb and index finger and weakness and atrophy of the thenar eminence (opponens, thumb abductor, and short thumb flexor) but *no* weakness of the intrinsics (spreading or opposing of the fingers) a nerve root cannot be blamed. The median nerve is the culprit with the probability of carpal tunnel entrapment rather than a cervical root involvement.

BIBLIOGRAPHY

Bhala, R. P., and Goodgold, J.: Motor conduction in the deep palmar branch of the ulnar nerve. Arch. Phys. Med. 49:460, 1968.

Brown, H. A.: Treatment of peripheral nerve injuries. Rev. Surg. 24:1, 1967.

Carpendale, M. T.: The localization of ulnar nerve compression in the hand and arm: an improved method of electroneuromyography. Arch. Phys. Med. 47:325, 1966.

Dabbs, C. H., and Peirce, E. C.: Causalgia treated with chlorpromazine hydrochloride. J.A.M.A. 159:1626, 1955.

Doupe, J., Culler, C. H., and Chance, G. Q.: Post-traumatic pain and the causalgic syndrome. J. Neurol., Neurosurg., Psychiat. 7:33, 1944.

Doyle, J. R., and Carroll, R. E.: The carpal tunnel syndrome: a review of one-hundred patients treated surgically. Calif. Med. 108:263, 1968.

Dundee, J. W.: Chlorpromazine as an adjunct in the relief of chronic pain. Br. J. Anaesth. 29:28, 1957.

Gilliat, R. W., and Wilson, T. G.: A pneumatic tourniquet test in the carpal tunnel syndrome. Lancet 2:595, 1953.

Hale, M. S.: A practical Approach to Arm Pain. Charles C Thomas, Springfield, Ill., 1971.

Homans, J.: Minor causalgia: A hyperesthetic neurovascular syndrome. New Eng. J. Med. 222:870, 1940.

Kendall, D.: Aetiology, diagnosis, and treatment of paraesthesiae in the hands. British Med. J. 2:1633, 1960.

Kopell, H. P., and Thompson, W. A. L.: Peripheral Entrapment Neuropathies. Williams & Wilkins Company, Baltimore, 1963.

Lampe, E. W.: Surgical anatomy of the hand. CIBA Clin. Sympos. 9: Jan. - Feb., 1967.

Magee, R. B., and Palen, G. S.: Tardy ulnar palsy. Amer. J. Surg. 78:470, 1949.

Marinacci, A. A.: Comparative value of measurement of nerve conduction velocity and electromyography in the diagnosis of carpal tunnel syndrome. Arch. Phys. Med. 45:548, 1964.

Marinacci, A. A., and Von Hagen, R. O.: Misleading all median hand. Arch. Neurol. 12:80, 1965.

Mayfield, F. H.: Causalgia. Charles C Thomas, Publisher, Springfield, Ill., 1951.

Mitchell, S. W., Moorehouse, G. R., and Kean, W. W.: Gunshot Wounds and Other Injuries of Nerves. J. B. Lippincott Company, Philadelphia, 1964.

Moberg, Erik: Emergency Surgery of the Hand, W. M. McQuillan, trans. E. & S. Livingstone, Edinburgh, 1967.

Omer, G. E.: Evaluation and reconstruction of the forearm and hand after acute traumatic peripheral nerve injuries. J. Bone Joint Surg. 50:1454, 1968.

Shaw, R. S.: Pathological malingering. New Eng. J. Med. 271:22, 1964.

Steinbrocker, O., and Lapin, L.: Reflex Dystrophy: Reflex Dystrophy in the Extremities. Rheumatic Diseases: Proc. of the 7th Int. Cong. on Rheumatic Diseases. W. B. Saunders, Philadelphia, 1952.

Steindler, A.: Mechanics of muscular contractures in wrist and fingers. J. Bone Joint Surg. 14:1, 1932.

Trueta, J.: Studies of the Development and Decay of the Human Frame. W. B. Saunders Company, Philadelphia, 1968.

Watson-Jones, R.: Leri's pleonosteosis, carpal tunnel compression of the median nerves and Morton's metatarsalgia. J. Bone Joint Surg. 31:560, 1949.

Watson-Jones, R.: Foreword to ed. 2. The Care of Minor Hand Injuries, A. E. Flatt. C. V. Mosby Co., St. Louis, 1963.

CHAPTER 3

Tendons: Diseases and Injuries

Pain and impairment of the hand can result from injury to, infection of, and severance of the tendons. As in other tissues of the hand, knowledge of functional anatomy is essential for proper diagnosis and treatment.

TENDON SEVERANCE

Severance of tendons results in loss of motion of the joints involved. Treatment is surgical after certain basic concepts have been observed. The decision of initial (primary) suture rather than secondary suture after intentional delay depends upon the site of the laceration and the function of the tendon.

Extensor Tendons

The extensor tendons do not usually retract after being severed, thus they can be sutured soon after the injury. The severed extensor tendon must be kept sutured for three to four weeks; therefore, the suture material that must be used should not be absorbable and should ultimately be easily withdrawn. Stainless steel is preferable as silk cannot be pulled through tissues after three weeks.

The ends of severed tendons, once they are approximated, go through various stages of healing. During the first two to three days, there is an outpouring of fibrin. By the fifth day this fibrin mass is invaded by fibroblasts which form fibrils which fuse into long threads. These threads merge into bundles which bridge the gap between the tendon ends. By the third week, edema and increased vascularity are decreased and there is a sufficiently strong union to permit traction upon the tendon. These factors are the reasons for three weeks of immobilization following tendon repair.

Tendons contained *within* a sheath, when severed, show more deterioration and heal more slowly than those without sheaths. The swelling that occurs within the sheath apparently obstructs venous return and impairs tendon nutrition and healing.

Adhesions which form around a healing tendon present a serious impairment to function after healing is complete. Numerous approaches, such as wrapping the tendon in cellophane, local or parenteral steroids, and insertion of tubules of various materials around the tendons, have been tried to prevent these adhesions. None has been effective to date.

The technique of suturing tendons is beyond the scope of this monograph but is well documented in the literature. The ends of the severed tendon must be approximated and after suture, the wrist must be immobilized for three to five weeks with 30 to 40 degrees extension with the fingers also extended. This position of immobilization for sutured extensor tendons violates the general principle of immobilizing the hand in the *position of function,* with the wrist slightly extended and the fingers flexed. Sutured extensor tendons, however, usually result in good function.

The extensor pollicis longus retracts a considerable distance. The site of division of this tendon should not be laid wide open in an attempt to find the proximal segment. Rather, a proximal incision above the wrist should be made. When the tendon is located there, it can be passed through its passage by use of a smooth probe.

Flexor Tendons

Suturing of a severed flexor tendon in so-called no man's land (Fig. 68), has an unfavorable prognosis. This is due to the anatomical arrangement of the tendons in this area. A sutured tendon usually swells and here there is no room for expansion. Ischemic necrosis results.

When a tendon is divided in no man's land, primary suture should be avoided. Primary care should concern the wound with tendon transplant undertaken four to five weeks after the injury. Primary suture of the severed tendon in this zone not only gives poor results but often interferes with ultimate graft procedure.

Flexor tendons severed distal to no man's land (the profundus tendons) can be primarily sutured. In this situation the distal portion of the tendon usually is surgically removed from the site of insertion and the proximal tendon stump attached to the site of the old insertion. Shortening as much as one-half inch of the reattached profundus does not interfere with the uninjured superficialis function.

Flexor tendons that are cut *proximally* to no man's land, especially

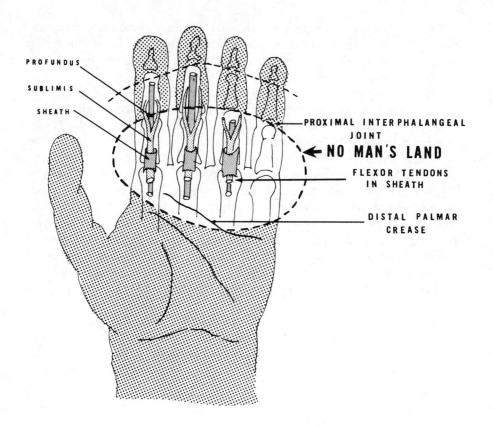

PROFUNDUS

SUBLIMIS

SHEATH

PROXIMAL INTERPHALANGEAL
JOINT

← NO MAN'S LAND

FLEXOR TENDONS
IN SHEATH

DISTAL PALMAR
CREASE

FIGURE 68. No man's land. This area represents the region where the flexor tendons (profundus and sublimis) are tightly enclosed within a sheath. Primary repair of tendons in this region is *contraindicated*. Merely suture of the skin should be contemplated. Primary suture between the two interphalangeal joints should be avoided because the tendon inserts in this region.

injuries at the level of the wrist, can be sutured with good functional results. Attempts to individually resuture tendons, for example profundus to profundus or superficialis to superficialis, usually result in functional failure. Usually only the profundus tendon is repaired. Because the profundus flexes the distal interphalangeal joint, good finger flexion results. When the superficialis tendon is severed, it is usually excised several millimeters from its attachment into the middle phalanx and allowed to retract. Suture of the cut flexor tendon of the thumb (flexor pollicis) usually gives good functional results.

After flexor tendon repair, the hand is immobilized for three weeks in slight wrist flexion with flexion of the involved finger or fingers. The *uninvolved fingers should not be immobilized.*

86

TENDON RUPTURE

A tendon may be ruptured from an acute stretch injury. The tendon normally is the strongest portion of the musculo-tendinous-osseous link and therefore seldom tears. Tear at its insertion occurs, with or without avulsion of the bone. Lesser stress may rupture a diseased or frayed tendon. Rheumatoid synovitis and fraying or moving over a rough bone fragment make a tendon particularly susceptible to rupture.

Mallet finger is caused by a forceful flexion injury to the distal phalanx during an activity in which the extensor tendon is taut, as in catching a baseball. The extensor tendon is torn from its insertion into the distal phalanx and in 25 percent of cases, a piece of bone is avulsed with it (Fig. 69). Clinically, the tip of the finger drops and extension is not possible.

Usually conservative treatment results in good function within five weeks by immobilizing the distal phalanx in hyperextension. There are numerous ideas regarding the best manner of immobilization ranging from casting the entire hand with the distal joint in hyperextension and the

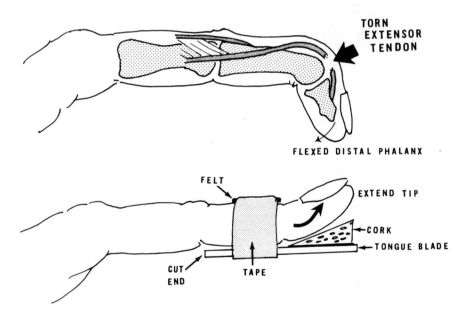

FIGURE 69. The mallet finger, rupture of extensor tendon to the distal phalanx. Forceful flexion of the distal phalanx may tear the extensor tendon from the distal phalanx. The end of the finger remains in a flexed position and cannot be actively extended. Treatment consists of immobilizing the finger with the distal phalanx in *hyperextension* for five to six weeks. The splint shown is a tongue blade reaching only to the middle phalangeal joint. A wedge of cork is glued to the blade and the finger is taped to the splint with a piece of felt inserted to protect the dorsum of the finger.

proximal joints flexed to merely splinting the distal joint as in Figure 69. By flexing the middle phalanx, the central extensor slip will pull the extensor mechanism distally and allow the tear to unite. The lateral bands will also be relaxed by this position (Fig. 70). If treatment is begun within 10 days of injury, it can be cast as shown in Figure 71 for five weeks followed by splinting of the distal joint for another four weeks. A short splint is worn for two more months to improve extension if there is pain, soreness, or functional impairment. If the proximal joints are stiff from previous treatment, this takes precedence in treatment and the flexed distal digit is ignored. Surgery is indicated when the residual functional impairment is unacceptable.

A fracture of the proximal portion of the distal phalanx, which clinically resembles mallet finger, must not be immobilized in extension as the resultant extended distal phalanx will have a greater disabling deformity. Open reduction of such a fracture is indicated.

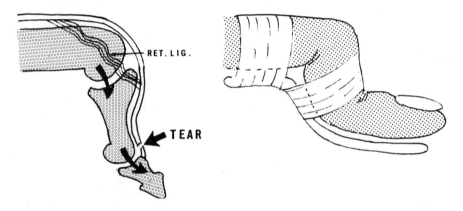

FIGURE 70. Rationale of treatment for mallet finger. Flexing middle phalanx and extending the distal digit permits the extensor tendon to unite. This position pulls the extensor mechanism distally and relaxes the lateral bands.

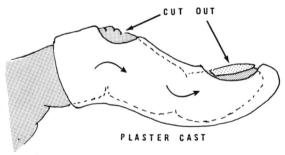

FIGURE 71. Plaster cast treatment for mallet finger. The cast holds the distal joint hyperextended and the middle joint flexed. The dorsum of the middle joint and the nail are exposed.

Extensor Tendon Rupture at Middle Phalanx

Rupture of the insertion of the extensor tendon into the middle phalanx, with or without bony avulsion, can occur from a direct blow or crushing injury. The injury may also attenuate the tendon permitting a subsequent forceful flexion to cause it to rupture.

Rupture of the middle slip of the extensor mechanism allows the lateral slips to move in a palmar direction (Fig. 72) below the axis of joint rotation of the proximal and middle phalanges (PP and MP in Fig. 72). Combining with the action of the flexor superficialis, the proximal interphalangeal joint flexes and the lateral slips extend the distal phalanx. Any flexion activity further separates the torn tendon preventing its union. Active extension of the finger also separates the severed tendon by applying tension upon the lateral slip.

Initially, in this tendon rupture, swelling and pain occur and all motion

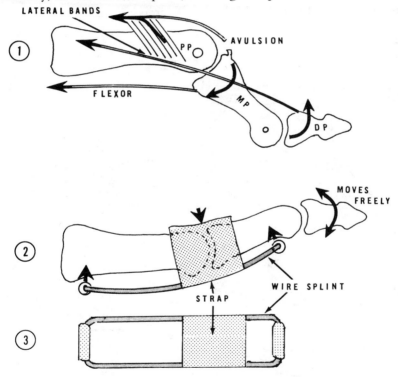

FIGURE 72. Button hole rupture, extensor tendon at middle joint, split treatment. (1) The avulsion of the extensor tendon, permitting the lateral bands to move in a palmar direction, pulling in a proximal direction. The flexor tendons now flex the middle phalanx (MP) and the lateral bands extend the distal phalanx (DP). (2) The splint is made of firm wire bent to extend the middle joint. The strap is inelastic. The distal phalanx is left free and motion is encouraged. (3) Dorsal view of the splint.

is restricted. Several days after the injury, the diagnosis becomes more evident. Flexion of the finger at all joints now becomes possible, but extension of the middle phalanx (middle joint) is restricted. If the middle joint is passively held in full extension, the spasm and retraction of the interossei prevent full flexion of the distal joint.

Treatment consists of splinting the middle joint in hyperextension and leaving the distal joint free (see Fig. 72). This splint can be made of firm wire fashioned in the shape of a paper clip and the finger held by a non-elastic strap. The splint is worn constantly for five weeks during which time the patient is instructed to *actively* flex the distal joint forcefully and frequently. When the distal joint can be flexed fully, it may be assumed that the intrinsic muscles are back in balance and that the extensor apparatus is reattached. The splint can then be removed. Surgical repair may be indicated (Fig. 73) when there is a bony avulsion or when the tendon tear has been of long duration before treatment is instituted. Normally, early diagnosis and proper splinting result in good functional recovery.

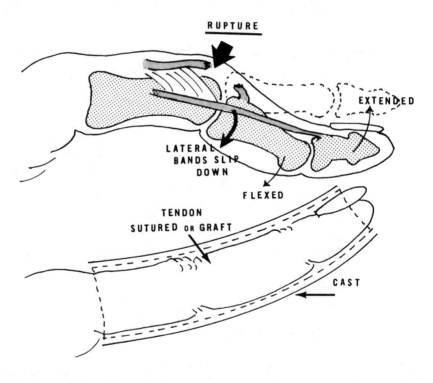

FIGURE 73. Extensor communis tear, surgical repair followed by plaster splint. The mechanism described in Figure 72 again shown. After surgical repair, the finger can be splinted as shown.

Extensor Pollicis Longus Rupture

The extensor pollicis longus tendon curves around the dorsal radial tubercle of Lister (Fig. 74), passes over the radial wrist extensors, and continues on to the thumb. At the point where the tendon angulates, wear and tear of the tendon occur. A Colles' fracture particularly can weaken this ligament. Rupture of this ligament results in the inability to extend the distal joint of the thumb and in weakness of extension of the proximal joint. Normally the tendon can be palpated when the wrist is extended and the thumb is abducted.

Primary suture of the two fragmented ends is *not possible* as it will neither hold nor function. Treatment requires surgical grafting of the severed tendon from a site proximal to the dorsal retinaculum to the end located at the metacarpal. It may be necessary to transfer the tendon of the extensor indicis. If grafting is done, a splint must be worn for one month.

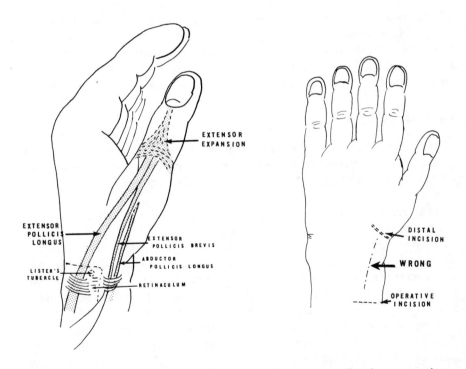

FIGURE 74. Rupture of the extensor pollicis longus. The extensor pollicis longus extends to the distal phalanx along a diagonal course. Its rupture results in loss of extension of the distal digit of the thumb, and some weakness of extension of the proximal joint. The ruptured tendon retracts considerably. End-to-end suture is not feasible, and grafting is required. Rather than extending the laceration, a proximal incision to locate the distal tendon must be made, and the graft is then passed through the canal with a smooth probe.

91

Rupture of Flexor Tendons

Flexor tendons rupture mostly when the tendons are diseased. Hyperextension of the fingers or forceful flexion against resistance is the usual history (50 percent). Many patients with this condition, however, do not give a history of injury.

Treatment of one or more torn flexor tendons depends upon the site of the rupture and the degree of disability as well as the underlying disease of the tendon. It is often best *not* to treat this type of rupture, as the treatment may cause more residual disability than does the rupture.

TENDON DISEASES

Tenosynovitis

Excessive repetitive movement or unphysiological stress of the tendon may inflame the tendon sheaths and cause painful impairment of motion. The symptoms include pain during any motion involving the tendon. The tendons are swollen and crepitation can be elicited during motion. The tendons most commonly involved are the dorsal extensors of the wrist, the extensor carpi ulnaris, and the long abductor and short extensor of the thumb (de Quervain's disease). Treatment consists of resting the part by splint or casting. Occasionally steroid injection is beneficial.

De Quervain's Disease

Stenosing tenosynovitis of the thumb abductors at the radiostyloid process is so prevalent that it merits special mention. This disease was named after the Swiss surgeon F. de Quervain who described the condition in 1895.

The tendons of the abductor pollicis longus and the extensor pollicis brevis usually move in the same synovial sheath (Fig. 75) that passes in a bony groove over the radiostyloid process and, from there, forms a sharp angle of as much as 105°. Synovitis results from friction between the tendon, the sheath, and the bony process. This friction occurs during pinching with the thumb and simultaneous motion of the wrist. During pinching, the abductor pollicis longus stabilizes the thumb.

Symptoms of aching discomfort are localized over the styloid process with radiation into the hand or up the forearm. Aching or pain is aggravated by movements on the wrist and thumb. Characteristic symptoms can be reproduced by flexing the thumb and cupping it under the fingers, then flexing the wrist in an ulnar direction which stretches the thumb tendons. Abduction of the thumb against resistance also can reproduce the symptoms. There may be tenderness over the tendon but crepitation is rare.

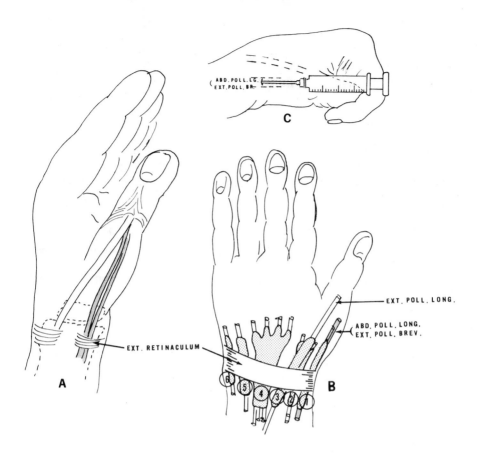

FIGURE 75. Stenosing tenosynovitis of the extensor pollicis brevis and abductor pollicis longus, de Quervain's disease. (A) The tendons pass over the prominence of the radial styloid process. The extensor pollicis longus tendon forms the ulnar border of the snuff box. (B) The six tendon sheaths pass under the extensor retinaculum. (1) and (3) are labelled. (2) contains the tendon of the extensor carpi radialis, (4) the extensor digitorum communis, (5) the extensor digiti minimi and (6) the extensor carpi ulnaris. Tenosynovitis occurs commonly only at (1). (C) The method and site of injection of steroids in this condition.

The pathology is an increased vascularity of the outer sheath that, coupled with edema, thickens the sheath and constricts the enclosed tendon. The synovial fluid of the sheath increases and turns a yellowish color. Fine hair-like adhesions may be found between the sheath and the tendon and the sheath may be thickened to two to four times its normal size.

Treatment requires immobilization in a padded half cast with injections of cortisone into the sheath. If, after four weeks of treatment, there is no relief, surgical decompression must be considered. Incision must not be longitudinal along the tendon sheath because an incision in this direction can cause a scar or keloid. A transverse incision followed by undermining the skin then a longitudinal incision of the overlying fascia and

93

the sheath will adequately decompress the tendon. Both tendons (abductor pollicis longus and extensor pollicis brevis) must be within the sheath or the decompression procedure will not relieve the symptoms.

Trigger Thumb

In this condition the thumb snaps as it flexes and may become locked in flexion or in extension. This situation occurs from thickening of the sheath or the tendon or both which prevents gliding of the tendon within the sheath. A nodule can form on the tendon which prevents the tendon from passing through the sheath at the metacarpal head.

Local injections of cortisone into the sheath may result in good recovery; if locking persists, excision of the thickened sheath is easily performed. The sheath is reached through a *transverse* incision at the crease over the metacarpal head (Fig. 76).

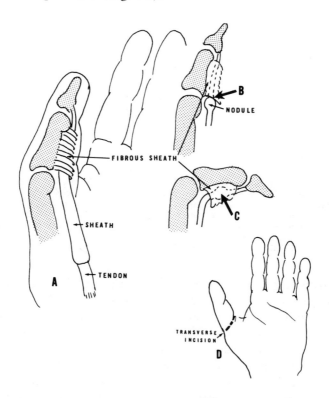

FIGURE 76. Trigger thumb, snapping thumb flexor. (A) The relationship of the flexor tendon within its bursa sheath covered by a fibrous sheath canal. (B) A nodular thickening of the tendon prevents flexion. (C) The nodule is trapped under the sheath and re-extension is prevented. (D) The site and direction of skin incision to decompress the tenosynovitis.

Trigger Fingers

Snapping flexor tendons or trigger fingers consist of a sudden snapping sensation of the finger during flexion and re-extension. Flexion is restricted; then the finger suddenly flexes to be locked in flexion and unable to be actively re-extended. This occurs mostly in the middle or ring fingers and is attributed to direct, severe, or multiple trauma to the flexor portion of the fingers. Injury pinches the flexor tendon and its sheath between the head of the metacarpal and the bruising object. The trauma may be acute and severe or repetitive.

The ligamentous sheath (Fig. 77) thickens. The tendon enlarges into a fusiform swelling and forms a nodule within its thickened synovium-lined sheath. The nodule moves within the ligamentous sheath until the nodule is too thick or the sheath too constricted, then obstruction occurs. The site of the nodule determines whether or not the finger can actively flex or is locked and cannot re-extend.

Cortisone injections into the sheath may relieve the obstruction. If this fails, a transverse incision proximal to the palpable nodule exposes the annular band which then is merely slit. Excision of the nodule invariably causes a new and bigger nodule to reform.

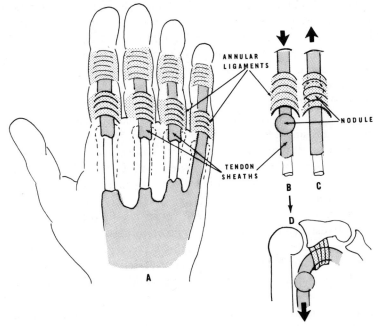

FIGURE 77. Trigger fingers. The anatomy of the flexor region. The flexor tendon within its synovial sheath passes under the annular ligament at the metacarpal head. (B) The fusiform swelling of the tendon plus thickening of the sheath proximal to the ligament. When it swells and gets in the position (D), re-extension (C) is prevented.

Dupuytren's Contracture

Dupuytren's contracture is a fibrous contracture of the palmar fascia with ultimate flexion contractures of the fingers at the metacarpophalangeal and proximal interphalangeal joints. The condition was first described by Clive in 1808, but Guillaume Dupuytren first described an operation for its treatment and his name has become associated with it. For no known reason the palmar fascia thickens and contracts. It is a disease found in Caucasian males in their fifth to seventh decades. There is no association with occupation, but there is a strong association with epilepsy and an increase in chronic invalidism such as pulmonary tuberculosis and alcoholism.

The palmar fascia covers the palm of the hand. It extends proximally as a continuation of the palmaris longus tendon passing distally into the fingers and ultimately attaching to the sides of the proximal and middle phalanges (see Figs. 32 and 33). In the palmar region the skin is firmly attached to the fascia by numerous fasciculi with scant subcutaneous fat.

The undersurface of the palmar fascia passes into the depth of the palm by perpendicular fibrous septa. These septa form eight longitudinal compartments alternately containing the flexor tendons and the neurovascular bundles and lumbrical muscles (Fig. 78). The palmar skin receives its circulation from tiny branches of the superficial volar arch (see Fig. 53) which penetrates the palmar fascia. As the fascia undergoes fibrosis, thickens, and contracts, it pulls upon the tiny fasciculi connected to the skin causing the skin to *dimple*. Further thickening of the fascia occludes the circulation and the skin atrophies. This explains the poor postoperative healing. The palmar fascia thickening involves the perpendicular septa and distally the longitudinal bands that pass over the metacarpal heads and attach to the base of the phalanges. As the fascia fibrosis contracts it forms nodules and the fingers develop flexion contracture. Stretching of the fascia by extension of the finger joints causes the involved longitudinally oriented fibers to react by contraction and further hypertrophy.

Symptoms usually consist of *painless* thickening of the palmar skin and underlying fascia with either dimpling or formation of nodules. The initial site is usually near the distal palmar crease (Fig. 73). Although any of the digits can be involved, the ring and little finger are the most common. Forty percent of patients have the condition bilaterally. Handedness is not relevant.

Flexion contracture gradually develops in the fingers at the metacarpophalangeal and proximal interphalangeal joints. Symptoms are functional disability and disturbing appearance but pain is rare. The fibrous band along the palmar aspect of the fingers with limited digit extension is characteristic.

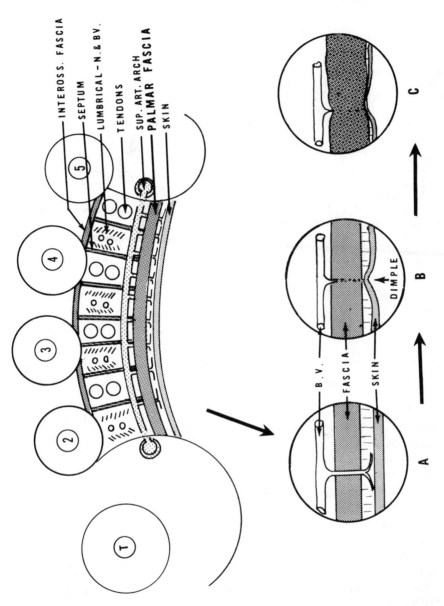

FIGURE 78. Dupuytren's contracture. The upper picture shows the normal anatomy of the palmar fascia. The palmar skin is firmly attached with little subcutaneous fat. Fibrous septa penetrate to the deep interosseous fascia and form spaces. These eight compartments contain the flexor tendons with the alternate compartments containing the lumbrical muscles and neurovascular elements. The skin receives its blood supply by vessels from the superficial arch which penetrates through the fascia. (A) An enlargement of the normal palm. (B) Thickening of the fascia constricting the penetrating nutrient artery. The skin puckers to form the characteristic dimple. (C) The fascia ultimately becomes markedly thickened and contracted and the overlying skin atrophic.

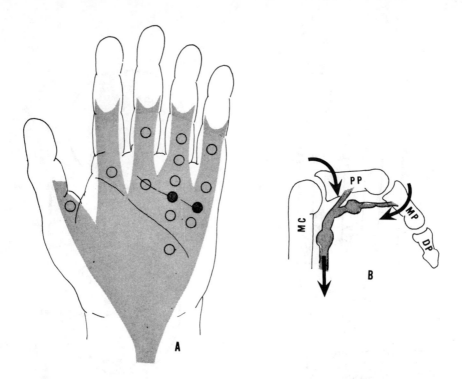

FIGURE 79. Dupuytren's contracture, site and mechanism. (A) The principal sites where nodules form in the palmar fascia. The fourth and fifth fingers are most frequently involved. (B) The fascial slips extend to the second phalanx (MP). When they shorten due to contracture they cause flexion deformity of the metacarpophalangeal or proximal interphalangeal joints or both.

Since hypertrophy is caused by stress, release of the stress decreases the fibrous hypertrophy. Release may be accomplished by merely excising the fascial bands—simple incision release of skin and fascia followed by skin graft insertion. The fascia that is incised is limited or confined to the palmar fascia and the contracted digit. The depth of the excision is limited to the more superficial longitudinal fascial bundles and transverse interdigital fibers. The transverse palmar hands are not involved and thus are not interrupted.

Preservation of skin blood supply, atraumatic dissection, closure without tension, absolute hemostasis, and early immobilization are the criteria of successful surgery. Contracture of the oblique retinacular ligament may occur from Dupuytren's contracture. This can be tested as illustrated in Figure 80.

Nonoperative treatment is being revived from Dupuytren's contracture. Injection of trypsin, alfa chymotrypsin, hyaluronidase, and lidocaine followed by forceful extension of the finger ruptures the skin and contracted fascia. Both of these ultimately heal with good finger range of motion. This nonoperative treatment is recommended in elderly patients or in those unfit for surgery.

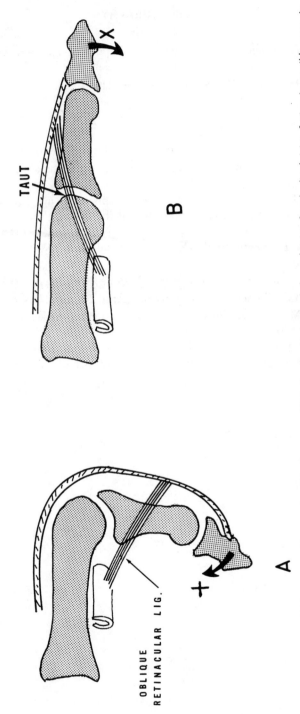

FIGURE 80. Test for contracted oblique retinacular ligaments. With the proximal interphalangeal joint flexed, distal joint flexion is possible even in contracted retinacular fibers; but with the finger extended, no distal flexion is possible.

BIBLIOGRAPHY

Bassot, J.: Traitment de las maladie de Dupuytren par exercise pharmaco-dynamic base physiologique technique. Gaz. Hop. 16:557, 1969.

Boyes, J. H.: Bunnell's Surgery of the Hand, ed. 3. J. B. Lippincott Company, Philadelphia, 1956.

Boyle, J. R.: Dupuytren's contracture. Etiology and principles of treatment. Calif. Med. 110:292, 1969.

Chase, R. A.: Surgery of the hand. 1. New Engl. J. Med. 287:1174, 1972.

Finklestein, H.: Stenosing tendovaginitis at the radial styloid process. J. Bone Joint Surg. 12:509, 1930.

Gonzalez, R. I.: A simplified surgical approach in the treatment of Dupuytren's contracture. Symposium of the Hand, Vol. 3. L. M. Cramer and R. A. Chase (eds.). St. Louis, C. V. Mosby Co., 1971; pp. 123-131.

Hueston, J. T.: Dupuytren's Contraction. Baltimore, Williams & Wilkins Co., 1963.

Luck, J. V.: Dupuytren's contracture. J. Bone Joint Surg. 41-A:635, 1959.

Palmborg, G.: Stenosing tenosynovitis. Ann. Rheum. Dis. 11:193, 1952.

Rhode, C. M., and Jennings, W. D.: Dupuytren's contracture. Amer. Surg. 33:855, 1967.

Skoog, T.: Dupuytren's contracture: With special reference to etiology and improved surgical treatment. Acta Chir. Scand. (Suppl.) 139:1-190, 1948.

CHAPTER 4

Fractures and Dislocations of the Finger and Hand

Fractures and dislocations of the fingers have frequently been ignored as trivial injuries yet have resulted in severe disability. The loss of finger function interferes markedly with the use of the entire upper extremity.

There are principles regarding the care of injured phalanges and interphalangeal joints that cannot be violated.

1. Immobilization must be instituted to relieve pain and permit primary healing. Active or passive motion will cause more, not less, stiffness. If tissues are torn, immobilization must be maintained at least for 10 to 14 days.

2. Immobilization must be maintained in flexion (Fig. 81). *No* fracture nor dislocation of a finger requires maintenance of *extension of all three joints*. The splinting of the entire finger on a tongue blade or straight metal splint is to be discouraged.

3. All digits that need not be immobilized *must* be *actively* mobilized. Only the injured part of the finger should be splinted and all other joints of the finger moved actively and passively. If one finger is immobilized in complete extension, it is impossible to fully flex the other fingers. Joints must be *actively,* not passively, moved and stretched.

4. Swelling must be avoided by elevating the hand and *actively* moving the shoulder, elbow, wrist, and fingers frequently through their full range of motion.

Fractures of the phalanges must be accurately reduced. This requires recognizing the exact site of fracture and understanding the muscle pull upon the fragments, then minimizing this deforming force (Fig. 82).

Interphalangeal joint sprains thought to be *simple* or *mere strains* often are subluxations or self-reduced dislocations with capsular tears or minor avulsion fractures. Recognizing this possibility is important since all

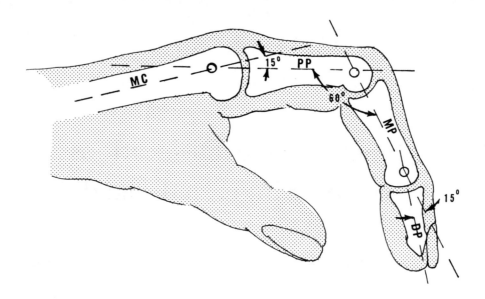

FIGURE 81. Position of immobilization of finger joints in treatment of fractures. Immobilization of the joints of the fingers in treatment of fractures is best done with 15° of the metacarpophalangeal joint, 60° at the proximal interphalangeal joint, and 15° at the distal joint.

sprains should be treated as dislocations or subluxations and should be splinted for two to three weeks in the flexed position then actively exercised. Painless functional recovery is thus likely.

Fractures of the phalanges distal to the metacarpophalangeal joint have the tendency to displace because of musculotendinous pull on the fragments. With the probability of fragment displacement, immobilization by traction is advisable. Traction is not used for reduction of the fracture but merely for immobilization of the phalanges in their proper position. Reduction is best done manually with the patient anesthetized or with an axillary block.

The duration of immobilization is *not equated with the time of healing.* Duration of immobilization is shorter than that of healing. Active range of motion exercises must be started before there is x-ray evidence of healing. This is usually within one to two weeks. Prolonged immobilization is as detrimental as is excessive manipulation.

Moberg has postulated comparative healing times (Fig. 83) claiming that the thinner distal portion of the phalanx is denser and less vascular and thus heals more slowly than the proximal portion and the proximal phalanx. The narrower distal portion on the middle phalanx heals in 10 to 14 weeks, the distal portion of the proximal phalanx in five to seven weeks, and the remainder of the finger in three to five weeks.

Open fractures should have the wound excised immediately under strict sterile technique and the wound covered as soon and as completely as

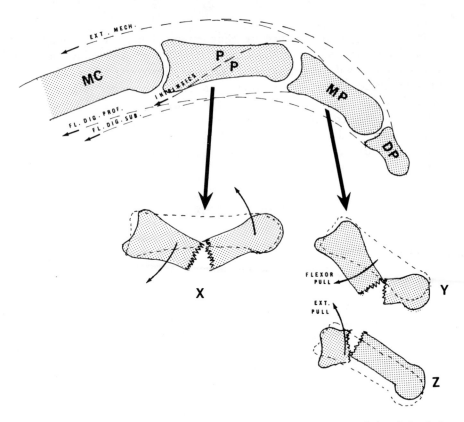

FIGURE 82. Phalangeal fractures, mechanism of deformation. Fractures of the shaft of the proximal phalanx (PP) bow in a palmar direction because of the pull of the intrinsics (lumbricals and interossei) which flex the proximal and extend the distal fragments. In fractures of the middle phalanx (MP) at the distal shaft (Y), the proximal fragment flexes due to the pull of the flexor tendons. In a fracture through the proximal shaft, the extensor mechanism acting upon the distal fragment causes dorsal bowing. Regardless of the site or direction of bowing, the treatment consists of traction, reduction, and casting in the flexed position.

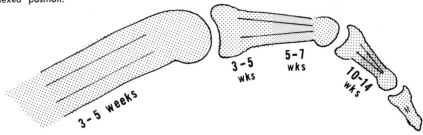

FIGURE 83. Fracture healing time. Bone relatively more vascular and cancellous heals more rapidly than denser bone. The former is found in the broader proximal portion of the phalanx and in the most proximal phalanx. The distal portion of the proximal phalanx consolidates in 5 to 7 weeks, whereas the distal portion of the middle phalanx takes 10 to 14 weeks. It is not necessary to immobilize fractures for these lengths of time. Modified after Moberg, E.: Emergency Surgery of the Hand. E. & S. Livingstone. London, 1967.

possible. Early, if not immediate, amputation of a severely damaged or crushed digit is desirable and indicated if it can be reasonably estimated that the finger will be permanently stiff, insensitive, and useless. Infection of a mutilated finger with resultant stiffness of the other fingers is best treated by resection of the infected finger thus preventing stiffness of the others. In children, amputation of a finger to avoid stiffness of the others should be delayed as permanent residual stiffness is not predictable. The maxim of early amputation does not apply to the thumb whose function must be salvaged as much as possible.

SPECIFIC FRACTURE SITES

Terminal Phalanx

These fractures usually heal without incident unless there is avulsion of the extensor tendon (baseball finger) or a subungual hematoma (Fig. 84). Treatment of a fracture associated with a baseball finger that

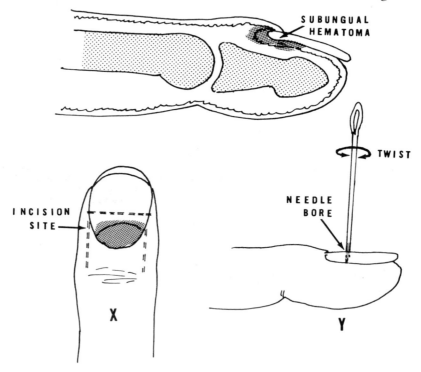

FIGURE 84. Evacuation of subungual hematoma. Upper figure shows the site of a post-traumatic hematoma. It can be evacuated by incising and elevating or removing the proximal half of the nail (X) or by boring a hole into the center of the hematoma with a needle heated to red hot and twisted through the nail (Y).

involves the distal joint should *not* include splinting in extension (the position for splinting the baseball finger) but rather splinting in the functional flexed position. A rigid distal phalanx in extension is more disabling than a flail flexed digit.

Subungual hematoma should be evacuated by lifting a flap of the nail or boring a hole directly through the nail (Fig. 84) with a red hot needle.

Middle Phalanx

Fracture here tends to bow the finger because of the pull of the flexor digitorum sublimis on the proximal segment (Fig. 82). Fracture of the proximal portion of the middle phalanx bows distally due to the pull of the extensor mechanism upon the distal fragment.

Treatment of phalanx fracture requires immobilization in flexion regardless of size and resultant deformity. If no displacement is evident, it is merely necessary to hold in a flexion splint, metal or plaster. If there is overriding or displacement or both, manual reduction is indicated and the finger is then held by traction (Fig. 85). Use of adhesive traction requires careful frequent observation to avoid slipping or skin damage.

Immobilization of the fingers in flexion demands that the fingers are flexed toward the scaphoid and not parallel to each other (Fig. 86). It is desirable that frequent x-rays are taken to insure that there is no bowing so that the tendons are not compromised.

Immobilization should not exceed three weeks before active mobilization exercises are begun. A night splint for protection may be desired when a callus is not apparent at the fracture site. A fracture extending into a joint gives a bad prognosis, and immobilization in a flexed posture is sought.

Metacarpal Fracture

Fractures at the base of a metacarpal are usually innocuous and merely need dorsal splinting for three to four weeks with simultaneous active exercises of the fingers and thumb.

Fracture of the shaft requires reduction by manual manipulation with plaster immobilization that permits active motion of the fingers and the thumb. After manual reduction if the fragments cannot be adequately held, then open reduction with the insertion of an intramedullary Kirschner wire may be desirable.

Fracture of the metacarpal neck requires manual manipulation for reduction followed by casting for three weeks, then active exercises (Fig. 80). Fractures of metacarpals especially with concomitant crush injuries should

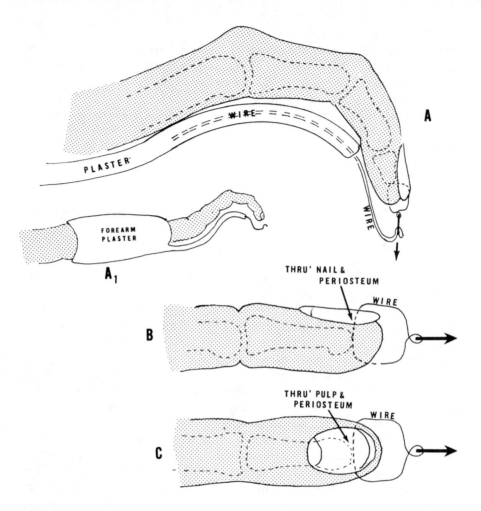

FIGURE 85. Fracture treatment with plaster traction. A braided stainless steel suture (0.08 mm.) or a traction pin can be inserted through the nail and distal phalanx periosteum (B) or through the pulp and periosteum (C) and traction applied by a wire incorporated into a flexed plaster cast. The cast extends to include the forearm A₁. Traction is used · to immobilize *not* to reduce the fracture.

never immobilize any of the digits nor the metacarpophalangeal joint. This is especially true of Negro patients who are more susceptible to scar or keloid formation. Active exercises must be instituted immediately and closely supervised. Physical therapy consisting merely of passive range of motion, whirlpool, and massage is ineffective. Patient participation in active exercises to use the full range of motion of each joint must be a full-time activity.

An Ace bandage applied to the swollen hand must be prohibited. A bandage that can be placed so as to constrict at the wrist or the proximal hand will only increase distal swelling. Chronic edema will lead to

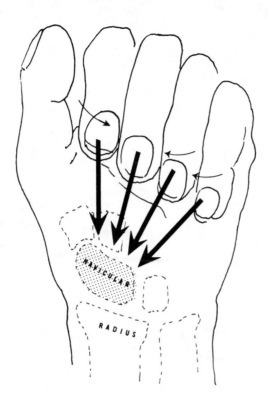

FIGURE 86. Direction of flexion immobilizattion in fractures of phalanges. The fingers normally flex across the palm in a direction towards the navicular bone. The axis rotation about the middle finger (arrows) cannot be incorporated into casts or splints.

fibrosis and a useless hand. During exercises and during much of the day, the hand is best elevated. A sling keeping the elbow flexed in attempting to elevate the hand is to be avoided.

Dynamic splints under watchful care in a well-motivated patient may decrease the digit contractures but they are not a substitute for frequent, *active* exercise.

Thumb Fracture

A frequent fracture site is the proximal metacarpal. These fractures (occurring mostly in men) result usually from direct blows to the thumb and are common in boxers. There are two major types of fractures of the base of the thumb: (1) that which does not affect the joint and (2) that which is associated with dislocation of the carpometacarpal joint (Bennett fracture).

In fracture of the base of the thumb without joint involvement, the

107

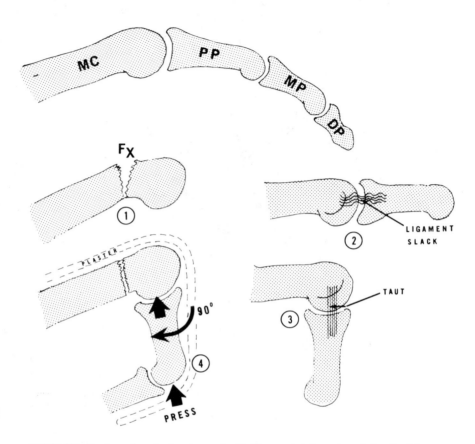

FIGURE 87. Fracture of neck of metacarpal. (1) The usual deformation of the distal fragment. (2) The lateral ligaments are slack when the proximal phalanx is extended so the fracture cannot be reduced in this position. (3) With the finger flexed, the metacarpophalangeal joint is immobile and the phalanx can be used to reduce the fracture which is then casted. (4) A dorsal splint applied for three weeks.

fragments are angulated dorsally and are frequently impacted. Reduction is accomplished manually with simultaneous traction and pressure over the base (Fig. 88) and casting which includes the forearm and maintains the thumb slightly *ab*ducted with the metacarpophalangeal joint flexed. The distal joint of the thumb is kept free and active.

A Bennett fracture occurs through the base of the thumb metacarpal separating a triangular fragment of the metacarpal. The metacarpal displaces laterally from the trapezium and moves upward (Fig. 89). The medial fragment is relatively unimportant. The metacarpal subluxes by sliding down the saddle-shaped trapezium, pulled proximally by the flexor and extensor tendons.

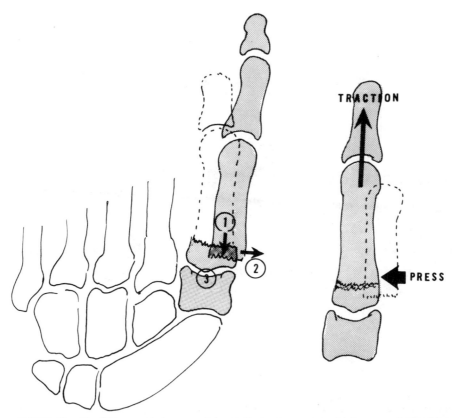

FIGURE 88. Simple impacted fracture of base of thumb metacarpal. Fracture of the base of the thumb metacarpal with impaction (1) and lateral displacement (2) but no involvement of the joint (3) is treated by reduction done with traction and simultaneous pressure against the distal fragment. The fracture is then casted.

Dislocation of the Base of the Fifth Metacarpal

Medial dislocation (in an ulnar direction) of the fifth metacarpal usually can be easily reduced; however prevention of redislocation by holding may require skeletal fixation. Lateral dislocation (in a radial direction) across the palm requires open reduction.

Dislocations of the index, middle, and ring fingers are unusual as these joints are relatively stable. Dislocation occurring either dorsally or towards the palm can be reduced by pressure upon the base with simultaneous traction. This is followed by a molded plaster cast for three weeks with simultaneous active exercises of the fingers.

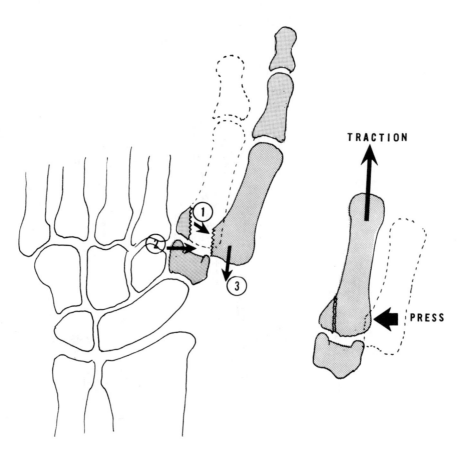

FIGURE 89. Bennett fracture of the thumb metacarpal. This is a fracture of the base of the thumb metacarpal with lateral displacement. (1) Fracture through the base. (2) Proximal dislocation. (3) The dislocation is aggravated by the pull of the flexor and extensor tendons. This fracture is reduced by traction with simultaneous pressure against the distal fragment. Prognosis is guarded because of residual instability and ultimate degenerative arthritis.

Wrist and Carpal Fractures

The most common fracture of the wrist is the *Colles'* fracture in which a fracture through the radius causes the distal fragment to be displaced *radially and dorsally.* A silver fork or dinner fork deformity results (Fig. 90). This fracture usually occurs from a fall on the outstretched hand. Sprains of this joint are rare, but displacement of the radial epiphysis is common in children. What may be originally considered to be a sprain with a negative x-ray should be viewed with suspicion and x-rays should be repeated in two to three weeks with oblique views to reveal concealed fractures.

Treatment demands complete correction leaving no residual evidence

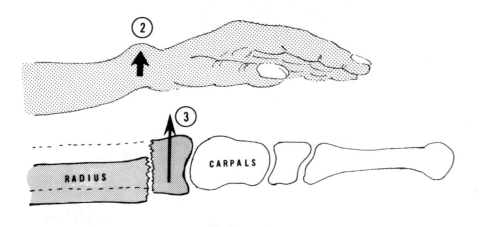

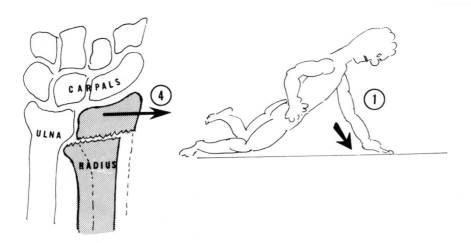

FIGURE 90. Colles' fracture. (1) Fracture usually occurs from a fall upon the outstretched hand. (2) Typical dinner fork or silver fork deformity noted. (3) The distal fragment is displaced backward (dorsally) and (4) outwardly (radially).

of a fracture displacement. Failure to reduce the dorsal displacement or the radial displacement will leave disfigurement and often limitation of ulnar-radial movement.

Reduction by manipulation can be done in one manuever but it is best done in two stages. The surgeon grasps the distal fragment (Fig. 91) with one hand (for example, the left hand for a right Colles' fracture) placing his thenar eminence over the radial fragment and the fingertips on the palmar side. The fragment is then pushed posteriorly. The opposite hand steadies the proximal forearm and permits traction.

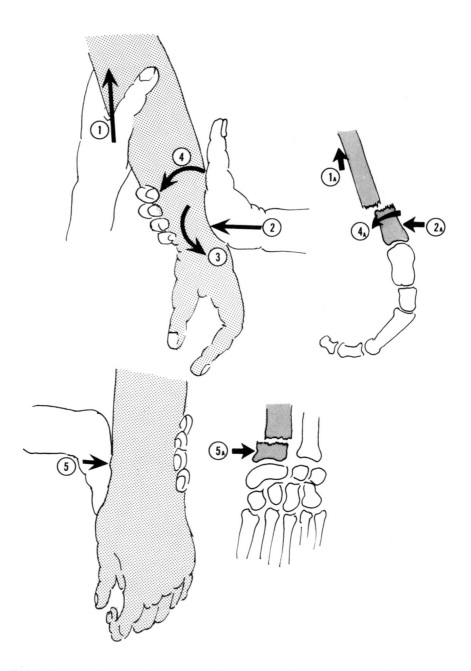

FIGURE 91. Reduction of Colles' fracture. (1) Traction applied in a proximal direction by immobilizing the forearm with one hand. (2) The thenar eminence of the manipulating hand presses the radial fragment posteriorly causing (3) ulnar deviation. As the fragment slips into place the forearm is (4) pronated. (5) A new grip is then taken and the fragment is pushed inward (ulnarly). The forearm is then casted in a carefully molded plaster.

The manipulating hand can exert some pronation while forcing the distal fragment into place. After the dorsal dislocation is reduced, the hands are altered and now the manipulating palm presses the fragment in an ulnar direction.

It is *not possible to overcorrect a displacement by manual pressure.* Only incomplete reduction can result. If the fracture is comminuted, complete reduction is mandatory and, in this situation, it may be necessary to compress the fragments between both thenar eminences of the manipulator.

After reduction, the wrist is immobilized in plaster applied while maintaining traction upon the patient's wrist by pulling on the thumb. The cast should extend from the upper forearm *to*, but *not including*, the metacarpal heads. The wrist should be molded before the plaster sets.

The cast should be sufficiently snug to prevent displacement but not so snug as to impair the circulation. In elderly people, the cast should be removed in 10 to 14 days and the wrist then placed in a more neutral position to prevent joint impairment.

It is imperative that active exercises be started immediately to assure complete range of motion of the fingers, thumb, elbow, and shoulder. These exercises must be started immediately after fracture reduction and done frequently, under daily supervision if necessary in the reluctant

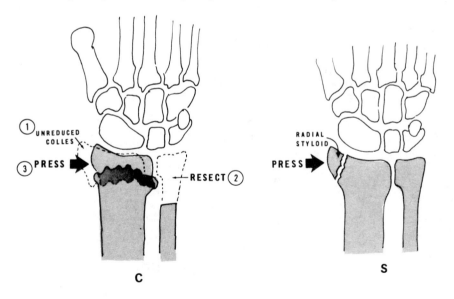

FIGURE 92. Treatment of an unreduced Colles' fracture, treatment of radial styloid fracture. (C) The unreduced Colles' fracture cannot be simply reduced after six to eight weeks. The ulna can be resected, then the radial fragment can be manipulated into position. (S) If the styloid process of the radius can be reduced by direct pressure it should be casted for four weeks.

patient. The arm should be elevated periodically to minimize edema. The cast should be maintained for four to five weeks. Earlier removal may permit displacement. A fracture that is unreduced after six to eight weeks cannot be simply reduced by manipulation but can be reduced by excising the distal end of the ulna (Fig. 92). Fractures of the radial styloid process can be treated simply by manually compressing the fragment if there is displacement, then casting for four weeks (Fig. 92).

A fall upon the outstretched arm causing forceful dorsiflexion of the wrist can cause a marginal fracture of the distal end of the radius which may be missed on original x-rays. A repeat x-ray may reveal the fracture. This is an important fracture that may deform the groove in which the tendon of the flexor pollicis longus runs. If this fracture is not recognized, reduced, and immobilized, an irregularity that can fray the extensor tendon may result. Immobilization for two or three weeks with avoidance of thumb movement is necessary.

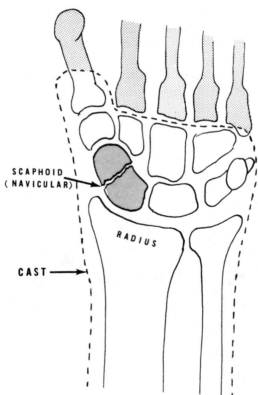

FIGURE 93. Fracture of the carpal scaphoid bone. This fracture is frequently missed on the initial x-ray and may require three views to reveal a hairline fracture. Suspicion is aroused by tenderness over the snuff box, swelling, and painful wrist motion. The fracture should be treated by six to eight weeks of snug plaster cast which includes the thumb metacarpal and extends to the carpometacarpal joints of the other fingers.

Injuries of the wrist demand x-rays taken in three planes. The x-rays should be looked at with extreme care, and repeated films should be taken as desired to ascertain the presence of a fracture of the scaphoid (Fig. 93). Scaphoid bone fractures *never heal spontaneously* without prolonged, uninterrupted immobilization.

Symptoms of fractures of the scaphoid are pain, tenderness, and swelling in the snuff box after a fall on the outstretched hand. Movement of the wrist is painful. X-rays must be taken in the anterior-posterior, lateral, and oblique views. Negative initial views *do not dispel* the diagnosis. If symptoms warrant, a diagnosis of fracture regardless of a negative x-ray treatment is justified. Only a negative x-ray three to four weeks after the fall is conclusive.

Treatment requires *rigid* plaster immobilization extending from the metacarpals to the elbow and including the metacarpal of the thumb. The thumb metacarpal should be fully abducted with the interphalangeal joint slightly flexed. After three weeks the cast can be removed and x-rays repeated. If then a fracture is revealed, the cast must be reapplied for a minimum of eight to ten weeks or when there is evidence of union by x-ray. Union is verified if the x-ray reveals *obliteration* of the fracture line. Immobilization is the only effective treatment. Surgical intervention offers little help.

CHAPTER 5

Joints: Injury and Disease

The study of joint disease and injury overlaps Chapter 4 by including dislocations as injuries to the soft tissues of the joints. Rheumatoid arthritis is primarily a disease of the soft tissue and ultimately manifests itself as joint deformity with pain and functional impairment. All are included in this chapter because of the similarity of structural changes and symptoms.

SPRAINS

Many sprains are momentary subluxations that spontaneously reduce. They escape x-ray detection and tend to be ignored or minimized. They should be diagnosed as *reduced subluxations* and, barring complications, treated by immobilization in a slightly flexed position of function for a period of two to three weeks followed by progressive active exercises. Limitation and swelling may persist for months following sprain.

In a subluxation, as in a complete dislocation, the capsule and collateral ligaments may be torn, but to a lesser degree. A capsular tear in which the head of a metacarpal or phalanx herniates may cause reduction to be difficult and the prevention of recurrence after reduction equally difficult. Effective treatment of this type of problem requires open reduction and surgical repair of the tear in the capsule.

Interphalangeal and metacarpophalangeal dislocations are usually caused by hyperextension injuries. Reduction is possible by traction with simultaneous slight flexion followed by immobilization of that joint in slight flexion (Fig. 94). Dislocation of the metacarpophalangeal thumb joint is the most common digit dislocation. The proximal phalanx usually displaces backwards (dorsally) and the head of the metacarpal may protrude through the associated capsular tear. The capsule and the flexor tendons button hole the head of the metacarpal and maintain the dislocation (Fig. 95). Open reduction and surgical capsular repair is necessary.

The fifth carpometacarpal joint is also a saddle joint and resembles the

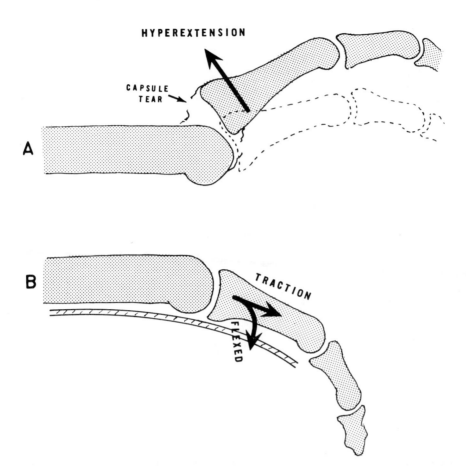

FIGURE 94. Subluxation of metacarpophalangeal joint. (A) The mechanism of subluxation from a hyperextension injury in which the capsule may be torn and the head of the metacarpal or the base of the phalanx can herniate. (B) Reduction is by traction and slight flexion with immobilization in slight flexion for at least three weeks followed by active exercise.

thumb metacarpophalangeal joint. Open reduction is usually necessary in a dislocation of the fifth metacarpophalangeal joint with a wire inserted to maintain the reduction. Degenerative changes ultimately occur, following dislocation of this joint, and these impair the cupping of the hand and thus prevent the formation of a good grip.

Carpal bone dislocations are common. A fall upon the dorsiflexed hand can dislocate the lunate bone in a palmar direction causing it to protrude between the capitate and the radius into the carpal tunnel (see Figs. 14 and 17). The flexor tendons and the median nerve are compressed causing swelling of the palmar area and limited finger flexion. Median nerve compression or carpal tunnel syndrome may result (Fig. 96). Reduction can be achieved by direct pressure upon the palmar aspect of the

117

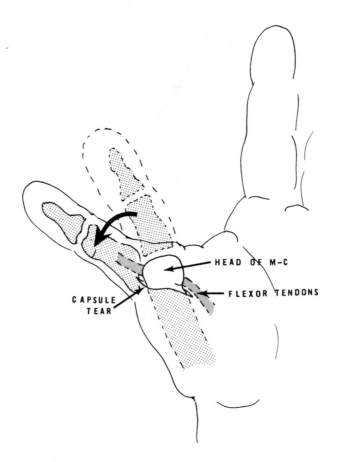

FIGURE 95. Dislocation of metacarpophalangeal joint of the thumb. The phalanx displaces backwards tearing the capsule. The head of the metacarpal protrudes through the capsule tear and gets button holed in the tear and by the flexor tendon passing behind the head.

lunate with simultaneous traction to the thumb and fingers. Healing then should be permitted with a cast.

RHEUMATOID ARTHRITIS

Rheumatoid arthritis is initially a disease of soft tissue, a disease of synovium. Half of the patients with rheumatoid arthritis have a disease of the tendons that are enclosed within sheaths. Tendons that are merely coated with paratenon do not undergo rheumatoid diseases. When they rupture, it is from mechanical abrasion of contiguous deformed joint structures rather than from rheumatoid disease of the tendons per se.

Rheumatoid disease frequently begins as a tenosynovitis that fails to be considered as a stage of rheumatoid disease until granulomatous synovium

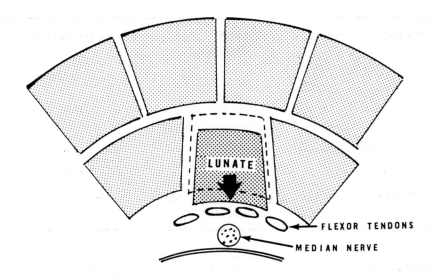

FIGURE 96. Dislocation of the lunate carpal bone. All the carpal bones by their shape, except for the lunate, dislocate dorsally. From a fall upon the dorsiflexed hand the lunate dislocates in a palmar direction causing swelling on the volar surface of the wrist and compression of the flexor tendons of the fingers and the median nerve.

invades the tendon causing it to weaken, lengthen, and even rupture. It is thought that the involved tendon ruptures because the invading synovium impairs its microcirculation. Although rheumatoid arthritis manifests itself early as a disease of the synovium, it ultimately invades all the periarticular tissues—the capsule, ligaments, tendons, and cuff tissues.

Treatment of the hand of the patient with rheumatoid arthritis is but one facet of the total care of a patient suffering from a systemic disease with an unpredictable variable course, duration, and residuum. Many contiguous joints of the upper extremity may be involved and these may affect hand function.

Care of the rheumatoid hand varies from initial care of the acutely inflamed hand to ultimate rehabilitation of the hand and fingers afflicted with severe structural changes. The acute inflammatory stage varies from mild aching and stiffness to severe and totally incapacitating pain, swelling, and limited movement. An acute fulminating onset is rare. The course is usually insidious and progressive, lasting several years. The acute stage usually subsides ultimately with residual destructive aftermath constituting the disability. The average duration of most acute inflammatory stages rarely exceeds five years.

The joints of the hand most frequently involved are the proximal interphalangeal and the metacarpophalangeal (Table 1). The acute

119

TABLE 1—COMPARISON OF THE RHEUMATOID AND OSTEOARTHROTIC HAND

	Rheumatoid	*Osteoarthrosis*
Joint Involvement	middle row and metacarpophalangeal	distal row
Wrist Involvement	usual	rare if ever
Tenderness	usual	rare or minimal
Swelling	soft of capsule and periarticular	hand bony

disease causes pain and swelling which restrict all finger movement. Such pain, however, causes most of the functional impairment by restricting flexion. Testing the patient's ability to make a fist does not significantly evaluate his disability. Loss of ability in handling small objects between the pinch tip-to-tip grip, manipulating tools of daily activities such as needle and thread, knives and fork, and even loss of the ability to handle a cane or crutches are far more significant in evaluating the loss of hand-finger ability.

Impairment of certain joints is more significant than others in causing disability. Loss of metacarpophalangeal and proximal interphalangeal joint function is far more disabling than is the loss of the distal phalangeal joints. Loss of flexion of the metacarpophalangeal joint of the ring and little finger prevents precision grip while using a knife and fork or small tools. Damage to the carpometacarpal joints of the ulnar aspect of the hand prevents full opposition of the fingers. Fortunately, when these ulnar joints are involved, they usually fuse in a functional flexed position.

Impaired thumb motion presents a major functional handicap. Damage to the carpometacarpal and metacarpophalangeal joints of the thumb prevents rotation of the thumb and impairs effective tip-to-tip opposition. If the thumb remains mobile but without rotation it may function by gripping side-to-side with the index finger which is a gross imprecise action. Loss of thumb abduction impairs the ability to fully open the grip for grasping large objects.

Treatment of the acute rheumatoid hand involves treating the in-flammation, swelling, and pain. In essence, treatment is directed primarily to the disease and secondarily to the hand. Rest is mandatory but is most difficult to accomplish as it must be local as well as general. Any movement of the rheumatoid hand, wrist, and fingers is structurally detrimental and painful, yet, all daily self-care activities, housework, and occupations demand constant hand and finger joint stresses.

Splints to rest the hand and fingers are usually ineffectual because they soon exhaust the patient's tolerance and cooperation. A kinetic splint can provide relative rest yet permit non-deforming motion. Such braces are usually cumbersome as well as difficult to adjust and maintain. Only rigid splints immobilize the affected joints but they deny adequate function. Static splints are usually used only for joint rest during the night or for brief rest periods during the day. At best they are a compromise because the deforming influences continue during unsplinted periods. Avoidance of any activity is best accomplished in a hospital environment but, except for brief periods during severe exacerbations, this is not medically, personally, nor financially feasible in a disease of prolonged inactivity.

Heat is soothing and may permit the patient to use his hand and fingers in painless *active* exercises. With heat, a skillful therapist may gently achieve an active and passive range of motion of most joints with little pain, discomfort, or residual distress. Application of ice often affords more relief than does heat, and its selection over heat depends on trial and the patient's choice. Physical therapy consisting mainly of local heat and unbalanced exercise may be more painful and harmful than willful neglect.

The type of exercise prescribed varies with the patient and must be modified according to individual tolerance. Active exercise with careful assistance or resistance or both by a therapist has value if there is no significant increase in discomfort and no lingering pain or tenderness attributable to the exercise. Isometric exercises, active muscle contraction *without* joint motion, will maintain muscle tone and decrease inflammation and edema.

In attempting to maintain or regain joint range of motion, the most important functional range must be sought. In the thumb, the most valuable range is that of rotation and abduction. Flexion of the ring and little finger metacarpophalangeal and proximal interphalangeal joints is as important as flexion of the proximal interphalangeal joints of the index finger. Once a joint becomes stiff, recovery is limited. An unstable joint may be more disabling than stiffness of a joint in a functional position. The hypermobile joint is further damaged by normal forces acting upon it. Damaging stress from improper alignment and failure to restrict unwanted movement can occur.

During the acute inflammatory stage of rheumatoid arthritis, surgical synovectomy has shown promise in removing the diseased pannus which ultimately causes joint destruction. If removed early, both the cartilage and the periarticular tissues are spared the destructive sequences of the invading pannus. The value, indications, and long range benefits of synovectomy as far as the specific joint involvement and the systemic disease manifestations are concerned remain unanswered.

Intra-articular injections of steroids combined with adequate physical therapy and bracing have value in certain joints but the long range value is limited. Injudicious repeated use may actually hasten joint destruction.

One of the common deformities of the metacarpophalangeal joints in rheumatoid arthritis is that of palmar luxation of the proximal phalanx in an ulnar direction. Although this motion is passively and actively possible in the normal hand, in the rheumatoid hand flexion of the fingers

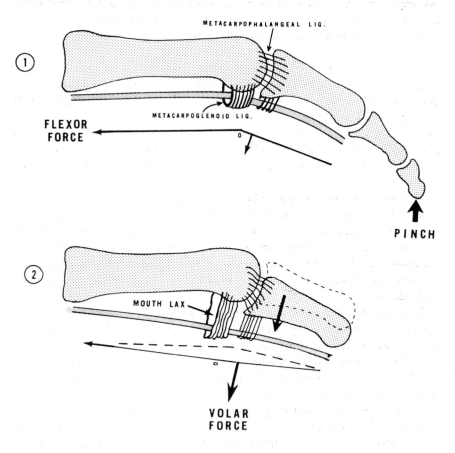

FIGURE 97. Mechanism of volar subluxation of metacarpophalangeal joint. (1) Depicts the normal pulley assembly that fulcrums the flexor tendons during a forceful pinch. The normal mouth of the tunnel is the flexor pulley. (2) In rheumatoid arthritis the tunnel and its mouth are frayed and elongated permitting the flexor tendon to move volarly causing the volar force to sublux the phalanx upon the metacarpal head. The metacarpophalangeal collateral ligaments are also relaxed permitting this subluxation as well as ulnar deviation.

always moves the proximal phalanx in an ulnar and volar direction and thus becomes a deforming action that must be avoided in the prescribed exercises.

When this motion is passively possible it implies a loss or diminution of the normal restraining tissues. When it is actively possible it indicates vector forces acting upon that joint. It must be assumed, therefore, from this excessive motion in rheumatoid arthritis that the passive deformity occurs first and that *normal* forces acting upon the diseased *joint* further the deformity (Fig. 97).

The collateral ligaments of the metacarpophalangeal joints are the predominant restraining tissues preventing ulnar and radial deviation (Fig. 98). There normally is ulnar deviation of the fingers because of the anatomic asymmetry of the metacarpal heads and unequal length of the collateral ligaments. When intact the intrinsic muscles reinforce the collateral ligaments.

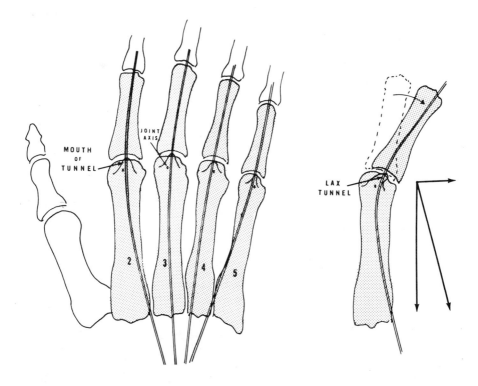

FIGURE 98. Mechanism of ulnar deviation (flexor concept). Normally the flexor tendons enter the tunnel of the flexor pulley which has a taut mouth. The tendons then veer in an ulnar direction. In index finger (2) and middle (3) the tendon passes to the ulnar side of the joint axis. The (4) and (5) tendons pass radial to axis. Normally the phalanges deviate ulnarly. In rheumatoid disease the mouth of the tunnel becomes lax permitting the flexor tendons to veer more ulnarly.

In rheumatoid arthritis, imbalanced musculotendinous pull against the collateral ligaments is considered responsible for ulnar deviation. The diseased intrinsic muscles are unable to compensate for the ligamentous instability. The radial collateral ligaments are elongated early in rheumatoid disease permitting ulnar deviation. In this situation the flexor and extensor apparatus become active deformers (Fig. 99) causing further palmar luxation in an ulnar direction.

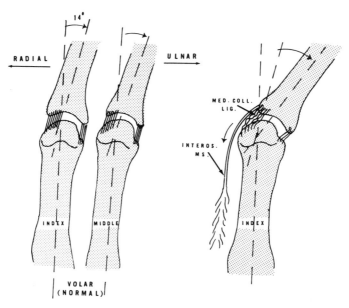

FIGURE 99. Mechanism of ulnar deviation of digits in rheumatoid arthritis. The normal hand finds ulnar deviation of the metacarpophalangeal of an average of 14°. This is most prevalent in the index and second middle fingers. In rheumatoid arthritis the collateral ligaments, especially the radial side, weaken and lengthen. The intrinsic muscles are unable to compensate for this deviation and ulnar shift results.

Treatment of palmar and ulnar deviation is difficult and requires prolonged tedious supervision when the disease is active. The dynamic ulnar deviation splint designed at the University of Michigan (Fig. 100) has proven to be effective.

Ulnar deviation may be cosmetically unpleasant, but not necessarily functionally disabling. Most grip functions are retained if flexion is retained. The greatest functional loss is extension of the fingers due to dislocation of the extensor mechanism. If ulnar deviation is marked, however, the tip-to-tip grip of the thumb and index finger may be lost.

Ulnar deviation of the little finger cannot be ascribed to the same mechanism since the flexor tendons bend in a radial direction at their tunnel mouths. One theory offered is that deformity occurs from the

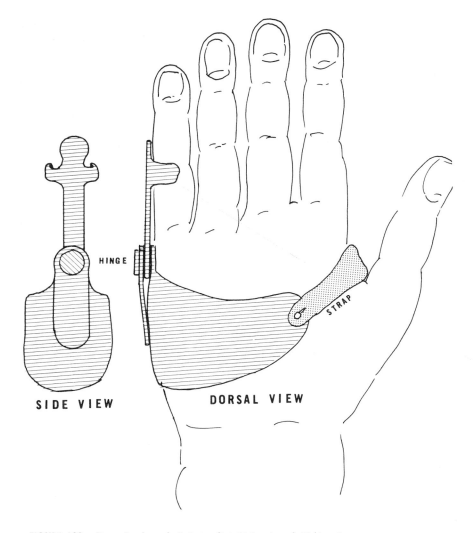

HINGE

STRAP

SIDE VIEW   DORSAL VIEW

FIGURE 100. Dynamic ulnar deviation splint (University of Michigan).

unopposed pull of the abductor digiti minimi. The hypothenar muscles attach to the ulnar side and are considered stronger than the palmar interossei and lumbricals on the radial side. Currently, the exact mechanism of ulnar deviation of the little finger is conjectural.

Disease of the tendons and periarticular tissues about the proximal interphalangeal joints may result in boutonniere deformity (Fig. 101). Because of thinning of the central slip of the extensor tendon, the lateral bands of the extensor mechanism dislocate to the flexor side of the joint fulcrum. This causes a flexion deformity of the proximal interphalangeal joint and hyperextension of the distal joint.

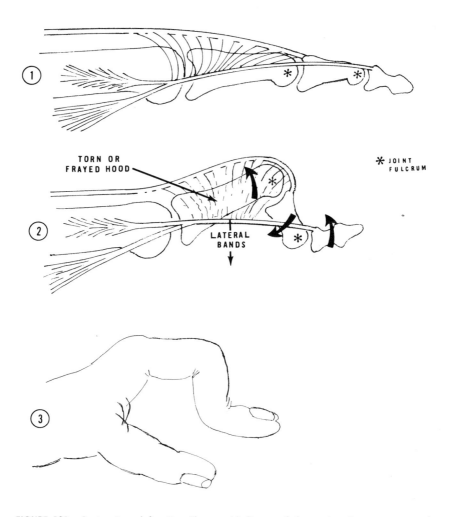

FIGURE 101. Boutonniere deformity. Rheumatoid disease of the tendon tissues causes weakening and tearing of the terminal portion of the extensor slip (hood) which normally holds (1) the lateral bands in place. As this weakens, the lateral bands dislocate in a palmar direction (2) and they now become flexors of the proximal interphalangeal joint and exert force sufficient to hyperextend the distal joint. The relationship of the lateral bands to the joint fulcrum is shown. (3) The appearance of the involved finger.

This deformity is difficult to treat. No functional splint is effective. Only a rigid splint can maintain the correction that has been gained manually. Surgical intervention leaves much to be desired as to functional improvement and frequently merely consists of severing the extensor tendon proximal to the distal interphalangeal joint and converting the digit into a mallet finger.

The extensor pollicis longus may be progressively frayed at the site where it passes around Lister's tubercle to insert into the distal phalanx of the thumb. This area of the tendon where rupture is most frequent is the area of poorest blood supply where the proximal and distal arterial vessels merge.

In rheumatoid arthritis with severe flexion deformity of the metacarpophalangeal joint, a treatment of creating an artificial insertion of the extensor mechanism to the base of the proximal phalanx to assist metacarpophalangeal extension is recommended (Fig. 102). This procedure may accomplish its initial objective but will *prevent* distal finger flexion and should not be considered without some caution.

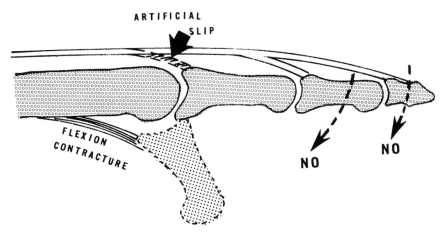

FIGURE 102. Surgical treatment of the metacarpophalangeal flexion deformity. The construction of an artificial slip to the proximal phalanx to assist extension also impairs flexion of the two distal digits. The flexion contracture is one of the disabling aspects of rheumatoid arthritis. If the extensor is anchored with fingers flexed (the proximal and distal interphalangeal joints), all long extensor action must be done by the intrinsics, which must be normal in insertion as well as innervation. This normalcy can hardly be expected in rheumatoid arthritis.

Rheumatoid disease of the tendons may cause formation of nodules within the tendon. These nodules may weaken the tendon and result in rupture or they may impair smooth passage within the sheath and result in snapping tendons also termed trigger fingers. This condition may be treated by steroid injections into the sheath or by surgical decompression of the sheath. Excision of the nodule, if extensive, may weaken the tendon.

Rheumatoid diseases may involve the muscle which in turn may disturb joint function. Inflammation and attenuation of muscle tissue is also possible from prolonged systemic steroid treatment. Inflammatory changes in the muscle result in spasm, later atrophy, and ultimately fibrous replacement and contracture.

Contracture of the intrinsic muscles causing secondary joint changes is exemplified in the swan neck deformity in which the proximal interphalangeal joint goes into hyperextension with simultaneous flexion of the distal interphalangeal joint (Fig. 103). In this condition if the metacarpophalangeal joint is passively held in extension, the interphalangeal joint cannot flex. Contracture of the intrinsic muscles extends the interphalangeal joint and prevents flexion of the distal joint.

This deformity can be averted by splinting to prevent or limit hyperextension of the proximal interphalangeal joint if utilized before contracture is manifest (Fig. 104). If the joint can be flexed, the split, worn

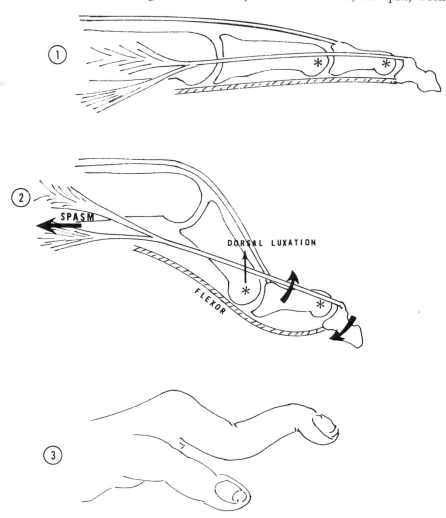

FIGURE 103. Swan neck deformity. Spasm then contracture of the intrinsic muscles (1) causes dorsal luxation (dorsal of joint fulcrum) causing hyperextension of the middle phalanx (2) and (3). Traction of the flexor profundus tendon causes the distal joint to flex. There is frequently flexion deformity of the wrist and metacarpophalangeal joint.

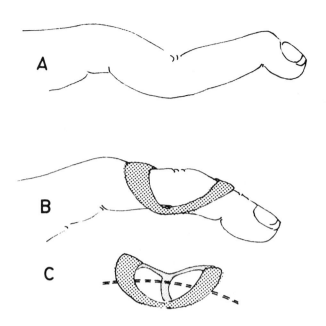

FIGURE 104. Splint for swan neck deformity. Before contracture and/or subluxation occurs, the swan neck deformity can be held or minimized by the simple splint shown in (C). This splint limits hyperextension of the proximal interphalangeal joint and permits flexion of this joint. Licht, S., ed.: Arthirtis and Physical Medicine. Elizabeth Licht, Publisher, New Haven, Conn., 1969.

day and night, permits the palmar plates and collateral ligaments to take up the slack. This splint permits finger flexion and thus maintains the integrity of the flexor mechanism. Discussion of surgical repair of this deformity is beyond the scope of this monograph.

Though swan neck deformity is most frequently caused by rheumatoid disease of the intrinsic muscles, there are other causes which also create deforming balance between flexor and extensor forces. (1) Contracture of intrinsic muscles causing flexion of the metacarpophalangeal joints and secondary proximal interphalangeal joint hyperextension are found in cerebral palsy and Parkinsonism. (2) Flexion contracture of the metacarpophalangeal joints or of the wrist can follow injury. (3) Weakness or overstretching of the long flexors causes stretch of the palmar glenoid ligament. (4) Ulnar nerve palsy can cause this deformity.

Deforming contractures and hand postures must be corrected or controlled or both. The diseased part must be rested, and disuse atrophy from excessively prolonged immobility must also be avoided. Prolonged immobility impairs the nutrition of cartilage and periarticular connective tissue as well as the viability of muscle.

Early immobilization permits the beginning of recovery and a reduction of pain. Active motion is indicated early, but a *full* range of motion may

129

be neither indicated nor desired. It is considered better to have a painless though limited joint motion or even a joint ankylosed in a functional position than to have an extremely mobile joint that is painful, unstable, and functionally inadequate.

Surgical improvement of the structurally deformed rheumatoid hand has definite value. Synovectomy has already been mentioned, but this alone will not correct existing deformity and dysfunction. If ulnar deviation is pronounced, the extensor tendons can be transposed over the joint towards the radial side to minimize the ulnar pull. In ulnar deviation of the little finger, the abductor digiti minimi may be divided and the extensor digiti minimi transferred to the radial side of the joint.

Reconstructive procedures vary according to the structural deformity and consist of division or deflection of the deforming tendons or the contracted muscles. Prosthetic devices are still in the experimental stage but hold promise. Fusion may be indicated when a painfully disabling joint laxity cannot otherwise be corrected and the patient can accept immobility of the joint as demonstrated by preoperative splinting. The specifics of surgical procedures are beyond the scope of this monograph.

OSTEOARTHRITIS

Degenerative arthritis or osteoarthrosis is a common affliction of mankind, known since antiquity and still eluding full understanding. Not having the serious portent of rheumatoid arthritis it nevertheless causes pain, cosmetic deformity, and functional disability to the affected hand. The label of "benign arthropathy of inevitable aging" has unfortunately denied proper treatment to many patients.

Many factors have been considered as playing a role in the disease. There are genetic factors dominant in women and recessive in the male. Hormonal factors affecting the progression of the destruction and the metabolism of cartilage predisposed to ultimate degeneration are enhanced by enzyme activities. Mechanical factors unquestionably are pertinent. The changes in the cartilage postulated to occur in this disease are noted in the superficial surface as a horizontal flaking. This occurs probably to a greater degree when the cartilage has been predisposed to insult by genetic, hormonal, and metabolic enzymic influences enhancing the adverse effect of trauma. Cysts form in the tangential layers that open into the joint surface causing rough craters. Enzymes such as hyaluronidase penetrate into the cartilage causing loss of chondroitin which changes the molecular composition of the matrix. Loss of cartilage elasticity results, synovial lubricants lose their viscosity, and further damage progresses until the destruction reaches the level of the subchondral bone. The subchondral bone successively fills in the denuded cartilage areas. Two incongruous opposing roughened surfaces with no interposed lubricant now exist (Fig. 105).

Degenerative joint disease is increasingly more common in older people with a marked increase in incidence during the sixth decade. In younger people it appears predominantly in joints subjected to recurrent stress such as the first carpometacarpal joints (trapeziometacarpal joint of the thumb).

Osteoarthrosis of the carpometacarpal joint is almost as frequent in its occurrence as are Heberden's and Bauchard's nodes, which are the osteophytes seen in the distal and proximal interphalangeal joints, respectively.

Osteoarthrosis of the proximal thumb joint can occur without evidence of osteoarthrosis in any other joint. Clinically, there is tenderness by palpation, stiffness, pain, and occasionally swelling over the joint. Crepitation is noted on movement.

Grip is impaired as a result of painful abduction of the thumb and weakness with atrophy of the thenar muscles. This condition is typically bilateral and more prevalent in women. A history of trauma cannot usually be elicited. Diagnosis is confirmed by x-ray, but other laboratory tests are unrewarding.

Symptoms, in comparison to other aspects of osteoarthrosis, do not respond to salicylates or indomethacin. Relief can be achieved by rest with avoidance of use of the thumb and immobilization using a leather or plastic splint. Local intra-articular injections of steroids (Fig. 106) give excellent but temporary results.

Surgery has its proponents and opponents. Excision of the trapezium relieves pain, but may result in grip weakness. Fusion may provide a pain-free joint, but solid fusion is difficult to accomplish and requires prolonged immobilization. Patients may then complain of the rigidity or the position of the thumb. The postoperative immobilization may impair motion of the other joints of the hand. Resection arthroplasty (excision of the trapezium) removes pain and provides mobility, however the joint becomes unstable and tends to subluxate. Recently resection of the trapezium with replacement by a silicone implant has been advocated (Fig. 107). Each patient's case must be judged on the severity of the symptoms and the desired functional residual required (Fig. 108).

Degenerative changes occur in the carpal joints and may cause severe disabling pain. Arthritis of the trapezioscaphoid joint may occur simultaneously with degeneration of the carpophalangeal joint of the thumb. These changes can occur in that joint alone. The flexor carpi radialis tendon passes near this joint so that underlying degenerative joint disease may cause synovial fluid to escape into the tendon sheath resulting in the appearance of a ganglion. This palmar ganglion is infrequent. Its relationship to underlying degenerative joint diseases can be verified by

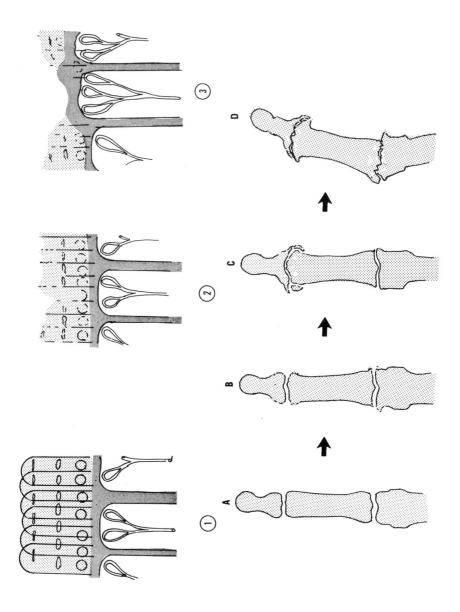

FIGURE 105. Natural history of degenerative osteoarthrosis. (1) Normal cartilage that through stress undergoes alteration of cartilage surface. (2) With penetration of synovial hyaluronidase into cartilage causing degeneration of the matrix. Collagen fibers erode as does the cartilage. Subcondral vascularity increases causing proliferation of bone into the denuded cartilage areas (3). (A) through (D) The typical x-ray changes from normal finger joints to early lipping of joint margins with gradual formation of periarticular ossicles and severe erosion with subarticular cysts and the obliteration of the joint spaces.

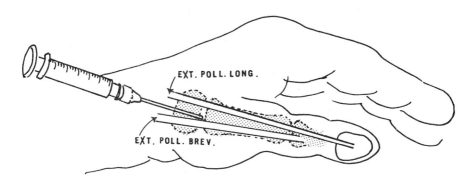

FIGURE 106. Treatment of arthritis of the trapeziometacarpal joint by steroid injection, technique. The joint can be felt medial to the elevation of the base of the first metacarpal. Flexing the thumb into the palm opens the joint more. The needle is inserted just lateral to the extensor pollicis brevis within the confines of the snuff box formed by the two extensor pollicis tendons.

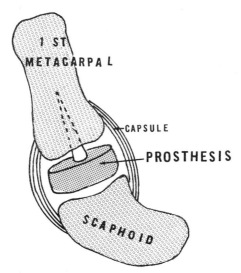

FIGURE 107. Silicone prosthesis for trapezium replacement. This prosthesis requires an adequate capsule and thus must be done early after resection.

an arthrogram in which dye injected into the trapezioscaphoid joint seeps into the ganglion.

General treatment of degenerative arthritis of any joint can be classified in its acute and chronic phases. In the acute phase, rest is imperative and must be specific, using a plaster cast or plaster splint if necessary. Active exercises should be avoided at first. Immobilization does not cause stiffness if carefully supervised, not excessively prolonged, nor instituted in an unphysiological joint position.

Local heat is valuable in affording temporary relief of pain, especially

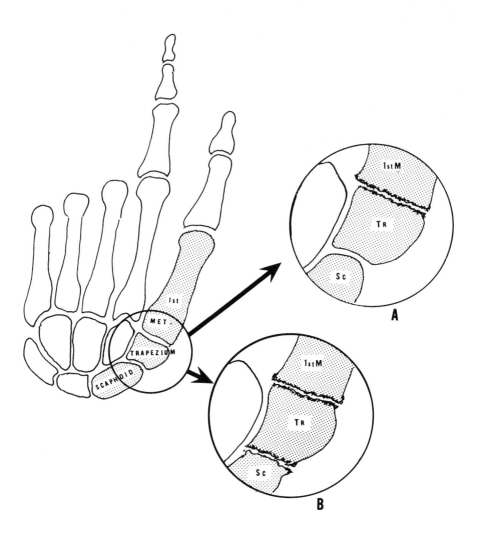

FIGURE 108. Surgical indications for arthritis of the trapeziometacarpal joint. Arthritis of the first carpometacarpal joint may require surgical intervention. These procedures consist of excision of the trapezium or fusion of the trapeziometacarpal joint. Excision of the trapezium gives relief of pain but the danger of resultant weakness of grip. Arthrodesis gives relief of pain unless there is arthritic change in the trapezioscaphoid joint (B).

when combined with oral anti-inflammatory drugs such as salicylates, indomethacin, or phenylbutazone. Muscular atrophy can be avoided or minimized with no aggravation of joint symptoms by instructing the patient in performing *active isometric exercises.* Gentle passive motion of the joints performed within warm water by a skilled therapist is soothing and beneficial. Intra-articular steroid injections are valuable, but must not be frequently repeated as there is evidence of joint destruction from repeated steroid injections.

Surgery for degenerative osteoarthrosis varies from arthrotomy with removal of damaged cartilage, to resection of damaged portions of joints, fusion, and reconstruction with prosthetic replacement. Careful team management should precede and follow surgical intervention for maximum benefit.

BIBLIOGRAPHY

Bender, L. F.: Prevention of deformities through orthotics. J.A.M.A. 183:946, 1963.

Bennett, R.: Wrist and Hand Slip-On Splints. In S. Licht, ed., Arthritis and Physical Medicine (Physical Medicine Library, Vol. 11). Elizabeth Licht, Publisher, New Haven, Conn., 1969.

Carstam, N., Eiken, O., and Andren, L.: Osteoarthritis of the trapezio-scaphoid joint. Acta Orthop. Scand. 39:354, 1968.

Duthie, J. J. R.: Evaluation of the patient with rheumatoid arthritis for corrective surgery. Arch. Phys. Med. 51:45, 1970.

Eaton, R. G., and Littler, W.: A study of the basal joint of the thumb: Treatment of its disabilities by fusion. J. Bone Joint Surg. 51-A:661, 1969.

Flatt, A. E.: The Care of the Rheumatoid Hand. C. V. Mosby Co., St. Louis, 1963.

Hakstian, R. W., and Tubiana, Raoul: Ulnar deviation of the fingers. J. Bone Joint Surg. 49-A:299, 1967.

Marmor, L.: Surgical Management of Arthritis. In S. Licht, ed., Arthritis and Physical Medicine (Physical Medicine Library, Vol. 11). Elizabeth Licht, Publisher, New Haven, Conn., 1969.

Moskowitz, R. W., Klein, L., and Mast, W. A.: Current concepts of degenerative joint disease (osteoarthritis). Bull. Rheum. Dis. 17:459, 1967.

Peter, J. B., and Marmor, L.: Osteoarthritis of the first carpometacarpal joint. Calif. Med. 109:116, 1968.

Shapiro, J. S.: Ulnar drift: Report of a related finding. Acta Orthop. Scand. 39:346, 1968.

Stillman, J. S.: The role of orthopedic surgery in the rheumatic diseases. Bull. Rheum. Dis. 20:568, 1969.

Smith, E. M., et al.: Dynamic ulnar-deviation splint. Arthritis Rheum. 7: 467, 1964.

Smith, E. M., et al.: Role of the finger flexors in rheumatoid deformities of the metacarpophalangeal joints. Read in part for Eighteenth Annual Meeting of the American Society for Surgery of the Hand, Miami Beach, Florida, Jan. 18, 1963.

Staub, L. R., and Chitranjan, S. R.: The wrist in rheumatoid arthritis. J. Bone Joint Surg. 51-A:1, 1969.

Swanson, A. B.: Disabling arthritis of the base of the thumb. J. Bone Joint Surg. 54-A:456, 1972.

Wynn Parry, C. B.: Rehabilitation of the Hand. Butterworths, London, 1966.

Zancolli, E.: Structural and Dynamic Bases of Hand Surgery. J. B. Lippincott Company, Philadelphia, 1968.

CHAPTER 6

The Spastic Hand

UPPER MOTOR NEURON DISEASE

An upper motor neuron disease affecting the upper extremity poses difficult treatment problems. Upper motor neuron impairment can occur in a child from prenatal and congenital insults such as anoxia, trauma, and vascular or infectious etiologies or, in the adult, from trauma, vascular occlusions, neoplastic or degenerative diseases, and cervical cord pathology. Each category varies in its severity, its progression, and its reversibility. The ultimate outcome depends on the cause, the patient's age, secondary manifestations of disease, the patient's mentality, and the effectiveness of prompt specific treatment of the disease entity.

Recovery of hand function may be favorable in a patient with a small, benign, and favorably-placed meningioma that is removed immediately upon discovery. Frequently, no treatment is needed for the hand after the lesion is removed. Evacuation of a subdural hematoma may also give favorable results. Hand involvement in multiple sclerosis may recover spectacularly as the disease undergoes spontaneous remission.

Upper motor neuron involvement of the upper extremity which persists after improvement of the primary cause, poses the serious problem of whether or not further functional recovery is possible. It can be stated candidly that the amount of functional recovery attributed to current treatment is meager. Rehabilitation of the spastic hand is more philosophical than practical, and more psychological than functional.

This assertion does not negate all treatment efforts nor designate all attempts to restore hand function as useless. Rather, it is a plea for realistic evaluation of the impairment, utilization of proven methods, and intelligent planning of treatment with concern for reasonable duration and frequency of treatment equated with sensible financial expenditure.

The problem requires long term management with continuous physical therapy, proper splinting, and appropriate surgery. Treatment of the child is more promising due to adaptation and inherent neural pattern development processes. *Retraining* of the insulted adult nervous system, however, is more difficult. Objective evaluation and scientific documentation of proposed treatments and the resultant recovery is needed. Better knowledge of the natural history of the impairment's recovery is necessary along with credited rather than glorified therapeutic concepts.

A rational evaluation of various modalities, standardization of techniques, and establishment of treatment frequency and duration must be undertaken. Recovery must be differentiated from maintenance of gained function, and a reasonable duration and intensity of treatment must be clarified.

HEMIPLEGIA

Wynn Parry has aptly stated the problem of the adult hemiplegic with the premise:

Anything more than a transient hemiplegia results in permanent paralysis of the intrinsics of the hand. Lumbrical and interossei action hardly ever return. There may be some coarse movement in the thumb, even some opposition, but controlled fine movements are not possible. All that can be expected of a hemiplegic hand is coarse grip and support.

This pessimistic prognosis in the adult hemiplegic is modified only slightly in the child's spastic hand. Functional utilization of improper motions in daily activities makes children more educable but, in reality, their improved function comes mostly through adaptation.

In the adult hemiplegic following a cerebrovascular incident, the extremity is flaccid from the immediate shock and gravity influences the position of the extremity. This flaccid stage may last for hours or weeks, although persistence of flaccidity for more than two weeks is a poor prognostic sign. Usually there is a gradual onset of hypertonicity of the entire upper extremity. This is a release phenomenon from cortical control resulting in loss of voluntary movements, increase of muscle tone (spasticity), increase in tendon reflexes and clonus, loss of cutaneous reflexes, and slowness of remaining voluntary movement. Neurological deficits cause the arm and hand to assume the spastic posture—pronated forearm, wrist flexed often in an ulnar direction, thumb in palm, fingers flexed at their metacarpophalangeal joints, and impaired extension of the digits.

Loss of *isolated* movements of the fingers and of all skilled motions of the hand is a severe impairment. There is loss of finger extension and wrist extension with the hand assuming a clenched fist attitude. The thumb is adducted and opposed into the palm and the elbow is usually flexed and the shoulder adducted. The patient is unable to voluntarily initiate the opposite of any of these positions. There is frequently a

138

sensory loss. The finer skilled movements usually suffer more than do the gross and less skilled movements. In essence, there is a predominance of uncontrolled flexor activity and the balance between flexion and extension is rarely recovered.

Poor dorsiflexion of the involved wrist while making a clenched fist may be a subtle sign of residual spasticity in a partially recovered or initially unrecognized hemiplegia. Aged patients who suffer a cerebrovascular incident may have their upper extremity assume a catatonic posture during ambulation yet be able to use their upper extremity fairly well while sitting or standing. After a mild cerebrovascular incident with resultant spastic hemiparesis, clumsiness of the finer finger movements is noted more often than is a loss of strength.

During the early phase of hemiplegia, when flaccidity predominates, proper positioning of the entire extremity must be initiated assuming that ultimately spasticity will occur. During this flaccid stage much damage may be done to the unprotected joint capsules of the shoulder, wrist, and fingers with resultant painful hand-shoulder syndrome, subluxation of joints, and excessive elongation of tendons and ligaments. Splints can be more easily applied at this phase than after the onset of hypertonicity. After the advent of spasticity, an uncontrolled, contracted posture leads to myostatic contracture, joint deformity, and muscular atrophy.

The position of the patient immediately after onset is influenced by gravity with the arm held close to the body and internally rotated, and with the elbow and wrist flexed. Proper positioning must be immediately established (Fig. 109) preferably by the nursing service during acute hospitalization or by adequately trained home-treating personnel.

Pillows are placed under the arm to position the upper arm away from the body with the shoulder abducted to 90°. The elbow is positioned at 90° flexion with the hand elevated and with pillows insuring partial external rotation. The wrist is maintained at slight extension by use of towels or splints (see Fig. 109) with the fingers kept slightly extended in a physiological position and the thumb in partial opposition and abduction.

During this phase *gentle* passive exercises should be performed daily with the objective of achieving the full range of movements of the shoulder and elbow, internal and external rotation of the arm, flexion-extension of the wrist, and full extension of the fingers and thumb.

Treatment during the acute phase consists of the prevention of contracture to make any spontaneous recovery unimpaired by contracture. Forceful passive exercises are to be avoided. The hemiplegic side also must be protected while the uninvolved side is encouraged to assume *all* functions. From the onset the concept must be accepted that the patient will ultimately perform all daily activities of self-care with his uninvolved extremity, and at best the involved extremity will be a gross helping arm

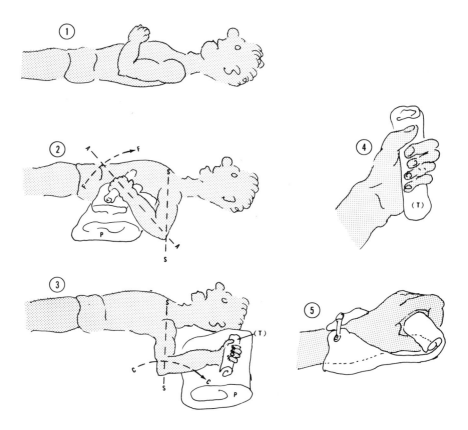

FIGURE 109. Arm, hand, finger positioning during acute phase of hemiplegia. (1) The usual position of the arm—adducted to the body, elbow flexed, wrist and fingers flexed, and forearm pronated. (2) Pillows are placed to abduct the arm to horizontal position (SS), forearm slightly externally rotated (FF), wrist extended as in (4) or (5). (3) When sufficiently mobile, the arm in the abducted position (SS) is externally rotated (CC) until resting upon the pillow (P). Wrist and fingers are kept in extension using a rolled face towel (T). (4) Rolled face towel is placed in the hemiplegic hand keeping the fingers slightly extended and the thumb abducted. (5) A towel folded and pinned as shown can keep the wrist extended and help keep the fingers from a clenched posture.

and hand and certainly not a painful and encumbering extremity. Any spontaneous recovery that occurs in the hemiplegic extremity will be considered a welcome addition.

As the prognosis of functional recovery in the hemiplegic upper extremity is extremely guarded and unpredictable, it is realistic for the patient to begin immediately using his uninvolved side for all transfer activities and self-care activities. As the uninvolved side may not have been the dominant, skilled side, much training may be necessary. Effort in this direction should be emphasized. Independence is achieved more quickly with this realistic attitude and the patient's psychological acceptance of his impairment is enhanced.

In the mildly involved hand, treatment should stress bimanual activities which should be done blind-folded to aid proprioceptive awareness. If a *mass* reflex motor response is invoked during an attempt to use a voluntary isolated motion, the patient should be guided to concentrate on separating the voluntary motion from the mass motion. Strengthening exercises of the weaker agonists should be performed. These usually consist of the opposition of the extensors to the hypertonic flexor muscles.

TREATMENT AND RECOVERY OF SPASTIC HAND

The spontaneous recovery of function of the impairment has not received significant study. Twitchell in his studies stated that initial movement occurred in 6 to 33 days after the stroke and occurred predominantly in the distal musculature. Van Buskirk found that functional recovery occurred in the first two months and *was spontaneous.* Bard and Hirschfeld in an attempt to prognosticate ultimate recovery found that many achieved no recovery, but those that ultimately achieved full recovery had initial voluntary motion in the first month and almost all expected recovery within two weeks. It was their conclusion that the extent of recovery was evident within the first month and maximum return of function within six months. Their studies unfortunately rated gross motions and were graded according to range of motion, strength, and endurance—not functional recovery.

From these reports there is good indication of the feasibility of intensive therapy for the first month after stroke with treatment continuing thereafter only if significant practical gain is noted. Continuation of intensive therapy after one month with no recovery only tends to maintain the joint range of motion, helps to retrain the good side, and aids the psychological outlook.

Many concepts and techniques of neuromuscular re-education have been postulated on the premise that the central nervous system can be trained to regain voluntary control of the hemiparetic extremities. Many claims of functional improvement are attributed to each technique, but ultimate functional recovery cannot be attributed to a specific technique as compared to natural spontaneous recovery or as compared to generalized exercise. Many hours of tedious exercises have been employed, utilizing well-accepted neurophysiological concepts and employing pathological reflexes, but none has been objectively evaluated as to its practical, functional returns.

Peszczynski rightfully questions the relationship between the concentrated learning of motor functions and the utilization of the substitution function. Do activities learned by intensive repetitive exercises ultimately become automatic unconscious movement? Does independent voluntary movement ultimately result from techniques employing mass reflex movements? In essence, can pathological reflexes be therapeutically converted into unconscious coordinated motor skills? Extensive clinical experience with these techniques compels the author to answer negatively.

The postulated progression of motor recovery in related developmental stages of cortical motor function as described by Brunnstrom, does not guarantee progression into the subsequent stage once a lower stage has been reached.

Neuromuscular facilitation techniques using mass patterns, stretch reflexes, summation, and pathological reflexes do not promise greater functional recovery than do simple active exercises. Motor activities are enhanced by sensory stimulation such as cutaneous icing and brushing. These practices have the immediate result of reciprocal relaxation and enhanced motor activity. However, improvement does not persist nor does it recur subsequently without more sensory stimulation.

Currently, neuromuscular re-education exercise techniques are experimentally attempting to clinically apply neurophysiological concepts verified in the laboratory animal. These concepts merit further study, but they are not justified for clinical therapeutic use since they require extensive technical skill on the part of the therapist. Such skill is not universally available nor necessarily desirable. Furthermore, these techniques require prolonged treatment which is not economically feasible nor justifiable and they also give unwarranted optimism to the patients and their families.

Physical therapy exercises are nevertheless justified and desirable in the treatment of the spastic hand. The weaker agonists, usually the extensors, should be strengthened. Repeated gentle passive and active stretching the spastic muscle groups should be performed daily. Brisk or forceful stretching of the spastic groups should be avoided as this increases the spasticity and is self-defeating.

Before any exercise or active therapy is undertaken, spasticity must be overcome or reduced. Removal or reduction of the spastic antagonist enhances greater voluntary function of the agonists. Cryotherapy can be of great value in reducing this tonicity. Total immersion of an extremity in ice or the application of ice over the spastic muscle groups reduces the spasticity. Cryotherapy temporarily permits greater function and facilitates treatment during the relaxation period.

Cold is best applied by using machine-made granular ice. This ice adheres to a terry cloth towel as it is immersed in the ice granules. The towel is placed over the muscle group for periods of 20 minutes. Three to four consecutive applications are recommended. Ethyl chloride spray is equally effective and simpler to apply, but it is more expensive.

Studies have shown that intramuscular temperatures remain normal during the ice application. Therefore it is postulated that the relaxing effect is mediated through skin receptors which in turn affect the gamma cells in the spinal cord. The skin must be cooled to below 20 C before spasticity decreases. Upon removal of the cooling agent, the skin temperature may elevate to 25 C without the return of spasticity. By this time, the intramuscular temperature has decreased and the muscle spindles are cooled. There are no verified contraindications to cryotherapy in the adult hemiplegia limb which already has impaired peripheral circulation.

In extremities with persistent, severe, and disabling spasticity, the spastic antagonist may be paralyzed or weakened by phenol nerve blocks which then permit greater use of the otherwise overbalanced weaker agonists. Once the motor point of the spastic muscle is located by electrical stimulation through a skin electrode, the exact motor point is more accurately located by injection technique (Fig. 110).

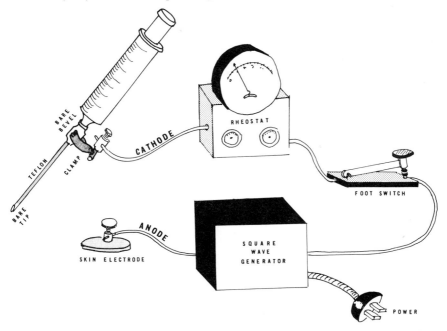

FIGURE 110. Procaine-phenol motor point injection apparatus. A syringe through which procaine or phenol solutions will be injected is connected to a 22 gauge 2 to 3 inch spinal needle that is coated with Teflon except for the bevel and the tip. A clamp which connects the cathode pole of a square wave generator is connected to circuit to modify the current which is reduced to the lowest that causes the muscle to contract. A foot switch permits freedom to the operator to manipulate the syringe. The circuit is completed by attaching a dispersing electrode to the same limb (anode).

The apparatus is a 22 gauge short bevel spinal needle coated with Teflon throughout except at its very tip and at the bevel. Teflon is better suited than is plastic or collodion as it permits autoclaving for sterilization and penetrates the tissues more easily.

A standard square wave generator cathode pole with a foot switch in the circuit, is connected to the needle bevel. The anode pole of the generator is attached to the same limb as a dispersing electrode. A rheostat within the circuit regulates the intensity of the current. Once the desired nerve is located by skin electrode, the specific site is localized by electrical current through the needle in which the minimum current causes the muscle to contract. Procaine solution 0.2 to 2.0 percent can be injected for relaxation from one to two hours. During this period it is possible to differentiate spasticity from myostatic contracture. It also permits therapeutic evaluation of the strength of the agonists and the availability of voluntary activity after release of the antagonistic spasticity. It may also permit a brief period of active physical therapy during the absence of spasticity. The primary value of procaine is to determine the exact site of injection and to decide the feasibility of following procaine with dilute phenol solution (1 to 3 percent solution in distilled water) which may give a period of relaxation of three to six months.

Mathews and Rushworth demonstrated the selective effect of dilute procaine upon the stretch reflex and subsequent studies substantiated the selective effect of more dilute solutions upon the caliber of nerves. A highly dilute solution of procaine was considered to affect the gamma fibers decreasing spasticity but not to inhibit alpha fibers. Nerve transmission remained. More recent studies refute the selectivity of phenol which allegedly acts like procaine. Phenol affects *all* size nerve fibers causing wallerian degeneration. The selectivity appears in the larger axons where regeneration of the affected nerve is slower. The smaller axons undergo degeneration and regeneration faster.

Phenol nerve blocks are not without undesirable complications. Causalgic states may result or persistent areas of anesthesia may remain. Skin sloughs have been recorded. Mild pain in the area of injection with tissue induration is to be expected but usually subsides in a few days with no adverse effect.

One current school of treatment of spasticity favors direct vision of the nerve to be injected and advocates direct vision chemoneurolysis as having fewer post injection sequelae and better results. The availability of a skillful and interested surgeon may influence this decision, but electrode needle injection done skillfully also has its advantages.

Surgical intervention of the spastic extremity using tenotomies or muscle belly releases is being prescribed more frequently. Spasticity of the shoulder, in which the arm is markedly adducted and internally rotated thus making the hand useless, may be surgically released by resection of the subscapularis muscle.

Boyes places great emphasis on contraindication of surgical intervention with spastic extremities, especially in children (C.P.). These contraindications include:

1. Insufficient conservative treatment preceding surgical intervention.
2. Generalized muscular weakness.
3. Severe lack of voluntary control.
4. Presence of athetosis.
5. Sensory loss.
6. Severe emotional instability.
7. Low mentality.

Keeping all these contraindications in mind, it must be categorically stated that most patients with cerebral palsy are not candidates for surgical intervention of the upper extremity. Rarely is an afflicted child a pure spastic or a pure athetoid. Rather they are mixtures of both due to diffuse brain involvement. Along with the presence of spasticity there is disorganization of the neuromuscular activity. Antagonistic relaxation fails on attempting voluntary motion so the flexors contract simultaneously with the extensors causing weakness and slowness of activity. Contraction of an agonistic also initiates reflex activity of the opposing muscle groups. Surgery does not alter this abnormality.

Pronation of the forearm intensifies all other hand dysfunctions. The pronator teres and pronator quadratus muscles causing this posture may be contracted and must be released before any other hand-finger surgical intervention can be considered. The spastic wrist is usually in a flexed ulnar-deviated position. Extension is weak if possible. The powerful flexor carpi ulnaris can be transferred around the ulnar border of the forearm and attached to the extensor carpi radialis to produce a strong wrist extension and increase voluntary supination.

Wrist fusion is rarely indicated and must be preceded by prolonged plaster cast immobilization before surgery is advised. Fusion *is* indicated if transfer of both the flexor carpi ulnaris *and* flexor carpi radialis to the finger and thumb extensor places the wrist in marked and functionless extension.

The spastic flexor muscles of the fingers may be attenuated by partial flexor tenotomies which then render the extensors relatively strong and unopposed. Release of the sublimis tendons is all that is necessary, but the released tendons must be attached to the proximal interphalangeal joints to prevent hyperextension deformity of the proximal phalanx into a swan neck deformity.

Before any surgery is contemplated, the procedure must be considered in relationship to the severity of the deformity, the ability and experience of the surgeon, the potential capacity of the remainder of the extremity, and the particular needs of the patient.

The deformity of the thumb in the spastic upper extremity is difficult to improve with bracing, splinting, and physical therapy, and causes marked restriction of function of the entire hand. Two deformities are usually present—thumb-in-palm attitude and the tightly adducted thumb. Both prevent abduction and open hand function as well as grasp and pinch motion. Spasticity of the adductor pollicis and the flexor pollicis longus are the major deforming forces.

Surgery consists of transfer of the flexor carpi ulnaris to the extensor digitorum to decrease wrist ulnar flexion and to extend the fingers, transfer of the flexor carpi radialis to the abductor pollicis longus, and release of the adductor and flexion contractures of the thumb. The web space may require a Z-plasty. In severe deformity, an arthrodesis of the first metacarpophalangeal joint of the thumb may be desirable, after a prolonged evaluation of preoperative splinting or casting.

In summary it may be stated that treatment of the spastic upper extremity does not promise much functional improvement with standard techniques of physical therapy, bracing, medications, or surgical interventions. A realistic program, however, must be undertaken in which maximum benefit is gained. The uninvolved extremity must be trained to its maximum for activities of daily function with the involved side as useful as possible as a helping hand. Ineffectual, prolonged physical therapy must be avoided since it places excessive financial burden on the family and the patient. Unwarranted enthusiasm with ultimate disappointment must be guarded against. Surgical procedures must be carefully evaluated to determine their possible benefit and to prevent any aggravation of further disability. Further research into therapeutic techniques, medications, operations, and modalities is necessary but must be conducted objectively, scientifically, and so reported before it is advocated as a therapeutic recommendation.

BIBLIOGRAPHY

Bard, G., and Hirschberg, G. C.: Recovery of voluntary motion in upper extremity following hemiplegia. Arch. Phys. Med. 46:567, 1965.

Boyes, J. H.: Bunnell's Surgery of the Hand, ed. 4. J. B. Lippincott Company, Philadelphia, 1964.

Burkel, W. E., and McPhee, M.: Effect of phenol injection into peripheral nerve of rat: Electron microscope studies. Arch. Phys. Med. 51:391, 1970.

Do It Yourself Again: Self Help Devices for the Stroke Patient. American Heart Assn., Inc., New York.

Granit, R.: Receptors and Sensory Reception. Yale University Press, New Haven, Conn., 1955.

Halpern, D., and Meelhuysen, F. E.: Duration of relaxation after intramuscular neurolysis with phenol. J. A. M. A. 200:1152, 1967.

Hartviksen, K.: Ice therapy in spasticity. Acta Neurol. Scand. 38:79, 1962.

Inglis, A. E., Cooper, W., and Bruton, W.: Surgical correction of thumb deformities in spastic paralysis. J. Bone Joint Surg. 52-A:253, 1970.

Kenny Rehabilitation: A Handbook of Rehabilitative Nursing Techniques in Hemiplegia. Kenny Rehabilitation, Minneapolis, Minn., 1964.

Khalili, A. A., and Benton, J. G.: A physiologic approach to the evaluation and the management of spasticity with procaine and phenol nerve block. Clin. Orthop. 47:97, 1966.

Knott, M., and Voss, D. E.: Proprioceptive Neuromuscular Facilitation, ed. 2. Harper & Row, Publishers, New York, 1968.

Mooney, V., Perry, J., and Nickel, V.: Surgical and non-surgical orthopedic care of stroke. J. Bone Joint Surg. 49-A:989, 1967.

Peszczynski, M.: Rehabilitation of the Adult Hemiplegic. Locomotor System, Fourth Annual Volume of Physiology and Experimental Medical Sciences, S. R. Mukherjee, ed. The Physiological Society of India, Calcutta, 1962-63.

Redford, J. B., Gelewich, G., and Jiminez, J.: Simple Splints, Principles and Techniques. University of Alberta Hospitals, Alberta, Canada, 1969.

Reynolds, G., et al.: Preliminary report on neuromuscular function testing of the upper extremity in adult hemiplegic patients. Arch. Phys. Med. 39:303, 1958.

Rood, M.: Neurophysiological reactions as a basis for physical therapy. Phys. Therap. Rev. 34:444, 1954.

Samilson, R. L., and Morris, J. M.: Surgical improvement of the cerebral-palsied upper limb. J. Bone Joint Surg. 46-A:1203, 1964.

Stamp, W. G.: Bracing in cerebral palsy. J. Bone Joint Surg. 44-A:1457, 1962.

Swanson, A. B.: Surgery of the hand in cerebral palsy and muscular origin release procedures. Surg. Clin. N. Amer. 48:1129, 1968.

Treanor, W. J., and Reifenstein, G. H.: Potential reversibility of the hemiplegic posture: Results of reconstructive surgical procedures. Amer. J. Cardiol. 7:370, 1961.

Twitchell, T. E.: The restoration of motor function following hemiplegia in man. Brain. 74:443, 1951.

Van Buskirk, C.: Return of motor function in hemiplegia. Neurology. 4:919, 1954.

Walshe, F.: Diseases of the Nervous System, ed. 10. E & S Livingstone, Edinburgh, 1963.

CHAPTER 7

Infections and Vascular Impairment of the Hand

INFECTIONS

Today with the newer broad spectrum antibiotics and the ability to determine drug specificity for a given pathogenic organism, hand infections no longer play the havoc they once did. The infected hand usually responds favorably and rapidly to early recognition and treatment. A trivial injury however, such as a small laceration or abrasion may spread into the fascial sheaths, tendon sheaths, or into the lymphatics and present a serious problem before antibiotic therapy is instituted. As in most infections, proper care requires incision, drainage, and specific antibiotic medication.

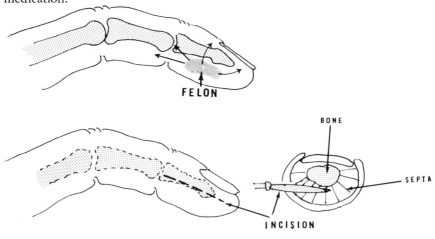

FIGURE 111. Felon, pulp abscess. A pulp infection may spread in the direction shown by the arrows—to the tip, to the dorsum, or retrograde into the distal joint or the flexor tendon sheath. The pulp is divided into compartments by vertical septa. Incision for a felon must cut across these septa and be near the nail to avoid later scarring of the sensitive tactile surface.

Felon

A pyogenic infection in the terminal pulp space is called a felon (Fig. 111). Pain and swelling of the terminal digit block the circulation to that digit and may result in ultimate necrosis of the bone diaphysis. A felon demands prompt and adequate drainage, best executed in a bloodless field.

The pulp contains many vertical septa between the bone and the skin which form numerous compartments. These can only be adequately drained by incising *across* the columns. The incision must be made near the nail to avoid scar formation over sensitive tactile pad surfaces. Care must be exercised to avoid cutting the distal flexor tendon. If a sizeable bone sequestrum has formed, it must be excised. Minor bone sequestra will regenerate if the epiphysis remains intact. The combination of early adequate incision, adequate antibiotic therapy, and removal of the sequestrum will give good results. Whenever possible, early referral to a hand surgeon should be made for definitive care.

Paronychia

Paronychia is an infection that occurs on the dorsum of the distal digit at the base of the nail. Initially there is redness, pain, and swelling. It is usually sufficient to elevate the skin fold over the base of the nail and incise into the sulcus along the side of the nail. If the infection has spread under the nail, it may be necessary to remove the base of the nail and pack under the remaining skin flap (Fig. 112).

Figure 113 shows the direction and site of incision for draining infections in the fascial spaces. Most infections are palmar but spread and swell on the dorsum of the hand since the dorsal tissues are looser. Most incisions for drainage therefore, are made on the palmar surface. The site of the infection is located at the area of maximum tenderness, local heat, and swelling. Usually infections are contained in the midpalmar space, the ulnar or radial bursal areas, or the thenar space. The various areas of localized infection are beyond the scope of this presentation, but several cardinal points must be emphasized.

When an infection spreads into the tendon sheaths of the second, third, or fourth fingers, drainage is accomplished by incising along the lateral aspect of the fingers. The incision must be made dorsal to the finger creases (see Fig. 113) to avoid cutting the digital nerves and arteries. Incision of the fifth finger is made on the radial side of the finger as there is less friction and trauma to that side of the little finger. For the same reason, incision is made on the ulnar side of the second (index) finger.

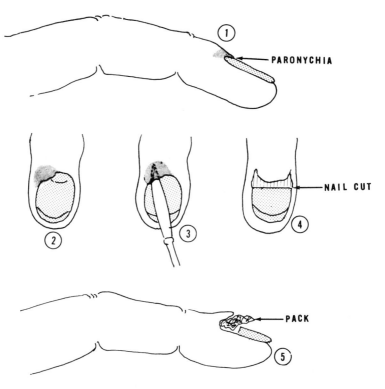

FIGURE 112. Paronychia. This infection begins at the base of the nail (1) and (2). If found early, it may be treated by elevating the overhanging skin by a sharp probe (3) and releasing the pus. If too severe, the nail may be cut as in (4), the proximal nail removed exposing the bed, and elevating and packing under the overhanging skin (5).

A midpalmar incision (Fig. 114) is made along or slightly proximal to the distal palmar crease. Once the palmar aponeurosis is penetrated, unusual care must be exercised to visualize and avoid injuring the digital branches of the median and ulnar nerves deep in the palm.

Drainage of a thenar abscess is done by incision on the *dorsum* of the web space between the thumb and index finger parallel to the margin of the web. If an incision is made on the palmar aspect of the thumb and thenar space, the proximal extent of the incision must be curtailed to avoid cutting the motor branch of the median nerve to the thenar muscles.

Infection that spreads into flexor tendon sheaths displays Kanavel's four cardinal signs—(1) the finger is held in slight flexion, (2) there is uniform swelling along the tendon sheath (as compared to localized swelling in the typical carbuncle), (3) there is intense pain on attempting to extend the finger, and (4) there is tenderness along the *entire* course of the tendon.

150

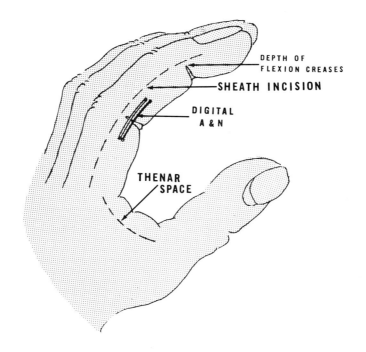

DEPTH OF
FLEXION CREASES

SHEATH INCISION

DIGITAL
A & N

THENAR
SPACE

FIGURE 113. Incisions for sheath infection. Incisions in the flexor tendon sheaths are made on the radial side of the fifth finger and the ulnar side of the second finger. The incision must be dorsal to the depth of the flexion crease to avoid the digital nerve and blood vessels. Infection of the thenar space is drained by a dorsal incision parallel to the margin of the web between the thumb and index finger.

It is apparent that proper care of hand infections requires combined use of local heat applications, elevation of the hand, proper use of specific antibiotics, resting the part in the physiological position of function, and incising for drainage. The latter requires extensive knowledge of anatomical structures.

Any surgery done on the hand must be undertaken under strict sterile conditions, preferably in an operating room and under ideal anesthesia. A bloodless field gives excellent exposure and is insured by wrapping the entire extremity with an elastic dressing, then using a blood pressure cuff inflated to 250 mm. of mercury, as a preferred tourniquet.

Unusual infections such as anthrax, gonorrhea, syphilis, tuberculosis, and various mycoses are suspected by their clinical appearance and must be verified by appropriate laboratory procedures. They respond to the fundamental care of all infections supplemented by specific antibiotic or chemotherapeutic drugs.

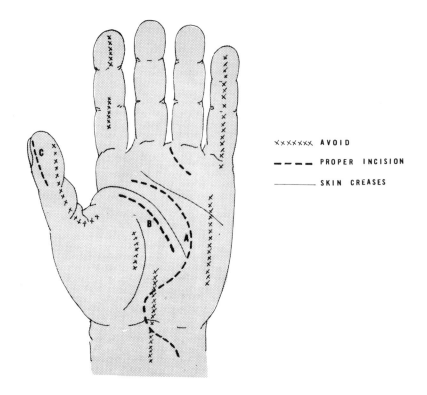

FIGURE 114. Site of incision for hand infections. (A) Incision for drainage of the palmar space between the median and ulnar nerves. The incision curves across the wrist crease to avoid contracture. (B) Incision for draining the thenar space; parallels the thenar crease. (C) Incision for drainage of felon. Transects fascial planes and avoids tactile surfaces. Avoid (1) cutting across creases, (2) over nerves and blood vessels, and (3) through tactile surfaces.

VASCULAR IMPAIRMENT OF THE HAND

Vascular impairment of the upper extremity can result from trauma, infection, or occlusive disease. The latter may variably evolve from embolic, thrombotic, neural, thermal, or mechanical pressure factors. The end result of vascular impairment is tissue necrosis with scarring, loss of muscle and tendon function, nerve impairment, and joint contracture.

Raynaud's Phenomenon

Raynaud's phenomenon is attributed to arterial spasm usually triggered by cold or emotional stress. It is most prevalent in women, around age 40, and is usually experienced bilaterally. An episode consists of sudden pallor of the fingers which may progress to complete blanching. The initial vasospastic period is followed by cyanosis, then a reflex vasodilatation in which the hand becomes hyperemic. Gangrene is rare.

Raynaud's phenomenon is a manifestation of vasomotor instability with abnormal sympathetic response to stress. This response may be secondary to numerous problems of the uncommonly recognized *cervical dorsal outlet syndrome* (anterior scalene syndrome, pectoralis minor or claviculocostal syndromes). Raynaud's phenomenon may be the forerunner of manifest-collagen vascular disease such as scleroderma. It may result from repetitive occupational trauma such as operation of a pneumatic drill. Regardless of the cause, nicotine is considered to be an aggravating drug.

Treatment should attack the cause and simultaneously support the susceptible patient with reassurance and prophylactic advice. Regardless of the cause, smoking *must* be discontinued. In inclement weather warm clothing and gloves must be worn. Handling iced objects must be avoided. Therapeutic drugs for the increase of arterial circulation such as nicotinic acid or priscoline have their advocates but give only temporary relief. In severe cases sympathectomy may be necessary.

Raynaud's phenomenon may result from mechanical neurovascular compression of the brachial plexus and the subclavian artery. Such compression may result from an anomalous first rib or a large cervical rib with or without contracted scalene musculature. Pressure upon the artery may cause thromboembolic disease with occlusion. Surgical exploration of the subclavian artery is necessary along with resection of the cervical or anomalous first rib.

The vasospastic disease of Burger rarely affects the upper extremity.

Disturbances Due to Cold

The impairment resulting from the exposure of the hand to extremes of cold varies with the extreme of low temperature, the duration of the exposure, the presence or absence of moisture and air movement, and the premorbid condition of the patient. Injury is more prevalent in a person with vasomotor instability, general debility, use of tobacco, and underlying vascular disease or previous regional trauma.

Chilblains is a mild cutaneous reaction from repeated exposure of dry skin to temperatures ranging from freezing to 60 F. The skin becomes red, warm, swollen, and itchy. There is no tissue destruction and treatment consists of avoidance of exposure with proper clothing. Soothing ointments may be used for subjective comfort.

Frostbite resembles first and second degree burns in its depth of tissue involvement. The first degree frostbite causes redness of the skin followed by desquamation. Second degree frostbite undergoes blistering followed by desquamation. Frostbite usually occurs from a brief exposure to extreme cold—below 20 F (-7 C).

Here the skin suddenly blanches, may tingle, then becomes anesthetic, and is brittle. Frostbite must be thawed immediately by immersion in a water bath of 104 to 109 F. A whirlpool when available is excellent treatment. When no hydrotherapy is available, the hand or hands can be placed under clothing into the opposite axilla. The frostbitten hand must never be rubbed and never be covered with snow or slush.

Early antibiotics should be started. The hands are then wrapped in non-adhesive gauze and placed in firm pressure dressings. Active motion of the hand and fingers should be avoided as the tissues are often brittle which causes the skin to crack. Sympathectomy and anticoagulation therapy have been disappointing.

The depth of tissue injury will determine the extent of residual impairment. Blisters usually occur within 24 to 36 hours and the skin blackens within 10 to 14 days. The exact mechanism of tissue destruction is currently unknown. Crystals form within the tissues, but the site and source of these crystals is obscure. As the frozen tissues thaw, lymph flow increases as does capillary permeability and edema results. Superficial blebs occur along with varying degrees of tissue necrosis.

Rapid thawing done *in the field* where the tissues may be refrozen should be avoided. Refreezing of tissues invariably ends in gangrene. Drinking alcohol to increase circulation defeats its purpose by the cooling effect of peripheral dilatation. The *general* body temperature must be elevated.

Occlusive Vascular Diseases

Occlusive vascular diseases may occur from embolic fragments originating from proximal thrombus formation as in rheumatic heart disease. Vascular anomalies and post-traumatic arteriovenous fistula may impair distal arterial circulation. Arteriography and appropriate surgery must be undertaken. Early referral to a hand surgeon or a vascular surgeon can salvage the impaired hand.

Volkmann's ischemic contracture results from vascular occlusion at the level of the elbow or forearm—most commonly the result of unexpected swelling in a plaster cast or from vascular compromise following a fracture or dislocation of the elbow. Other forms of trauma may cause this condition such as fractures of the forearm bones, hematomas from penetrating wounds, prolonged application of tourniquets, or even prolonged pressure upon the forearm during an alcoholic stupor.

Pressure mostly affects the flexor compartment of the forearm due to its peculiar anatomical structure. The compartment is tightly bound at

154

all its attachments and cannot expand to accommodate increased internal pressure. Pressure within this compartment from edema, venous congestion, or hemorrhage causes ischemic muscle, tendon, and nerve tissue necrosis.

The onset may be catastrophically abrupt with sudden painful swelling and discoloration of the forearm and hand. Cyanosis, coldness, and numbness are noted early. If pressure persists there may be necrosis of the flexors of the wrist and hand. The extensors are usually spared. The median and ulnar nerves are frequently involved but the radial nerve escapes entrapment.

The resultant deformity from this ischemic contracture is hyperextension of the metacarpophalangeal joints (due to unopposed extensors) and flexion contracture of the interphalangeal and wrist joints due to the contracted flexor muscles. The forearm is atrophic and a typical median-ulnar nerve hand results.

The best treatment is prevention. A constrictive cast must be released as soon as it is recognized. Elbow fractures or dislocations or both must be promptly and properly reduced. When done expeditiously, these measures usually insure proper circulation.

When circulation appears compromised from significant swelling of the forearm, pressure should be relieved by splitting the muscle fascia along the full length of the muscle bellies. The incision should be allowed to gape. The incision should angle at the bend of the elbow and all the major blood vessels should be viewed and freed from any obstruction. A skin graft should then cover the incision to avoid direct, open exposure of the underlying muscles. The arm and hand should be elevated and the fingers and wrist splinted in a physiological position. Early sympathectomy improves the circulation.

Any hand impairment resulting from ischemic contracture should be treated extensively by conservative measures before constructive surgery is contemplated. Serial stretch splints to extend the deforming contractures should be applied and changed frequently as increased range of motion is gained. These should be used for several months exercising care to protect the skin from unrelieved pressure. Physical therapy consisting of active and passive exercises supplemented by occupational therapy must be continued throughout the period of splinting and after the splinting has achieved its ultimate gains. This type of therapy should be instituted preoperatively and postoperatively, once reconstructive surgery is contemplated.

Vascular impairment of the hand also includes Sudeck's atrophy, reflex sympathetic dystrophy, hand shoulder syndrome, minor and major causalgias, and so forth. These topics have been covered in previous chapters.

GLOMUS TUMORS OF THE HAND

The glomus tumor is a tiny subungual painful tumor. The normal glomus is essentially an arteriovenous anastomosis without an intermediary capillary bed. The tumor is a "caricature" of the normal neuromyoarterial glomus with hypertrophy of the normal glomus elements. Myelinated and unmyelinated nerve fibers terminate within the glomus (Fig. 115). Grossly the tumor is soft, and pink or purple, with defined elongated mass the size of a grain of rice.

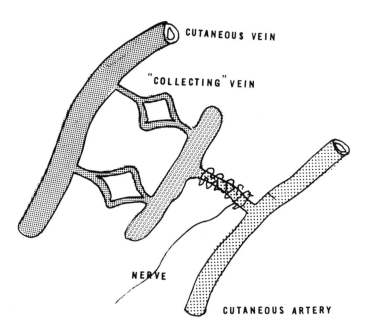

FIGURE 115. Glomus Tumor. The tumor is an abnormal connection between a cutaneous artery and vein in which there is swelling and thus irritation of the sensory unmyelineated nerve of the collecting arterioles.

The symptoms of a glomus tumor are pain, tenderness, and external sensitivity to temperature (cold more than heat). The mass (glomus) becomes visible or palpable after a considerable period of time, so symptoms can be present long before it is evident. When the tumor becomes visible it may be a blue spot in the subungual region, and there may be deforming ridges in the nail with the lesion being exquisitely tender. Subjectively the pain is termed "lancinating."

Treatment is complete surgical removal. It may be necessary to completely remove the nail, shell out the lesion meticulously, and currette down to bleeding bone.

BIBLIOGRAPHY

Allen, E. V., and Brown, G. E.: Raynaud's disease: A clinical study of 147 cases. J. A. M. A. 99:1472, 1932.

Boyes, J. H.: Bunnel's Surgery of the Hand, ed. 4. J. B. Lippincott Company, Philadelphia, 1964.

Carroll, R. E., and Berman, A. T.: Glomus tumors of the hand. J. Bone Joint Surg. 54-A:697, 1972.

Lampe, E. W.: Surgical anatomy of the hand. Clin. Sympos. vol. 9, 1957.

Murray, A. R.: The management of the infected hand: Based on clinical investigation of 513 cases. Med. J. Aust. 1:619, 1951.

Swinton, N. W., et al.: Unilateral Raynaud's phenomenon caused by cervical-first rib anomalies. Amer. J. Med. 48:404, 1970.

Wilkinson, J. L.: The anatomy of an oblique proximal septum of the pulp space. Brit. J. Surg. 38:454, 1950-51.

CHAPTER 8

Splinting the Hand

Proper splinting requires evaluation of impaired hand function then determination of the exact part to be splinted and the specific objective of the splinting. The objective sought by splinting determines whether the splint is to be static or dynamic and also specifies the duration and frequency of its application.

Construction of the splint requires imagination on the part of the prescriber or the orthotist. Patterns and molds are guide lines and should be modified to meet the special problem. Materials available are numerous and constantly changing. It behooves a frequent user of splinting materials and techniques to become familiar and adept with a special material and then improve his technique while employing new materials as they become available.

Splints should be specific but simple to apply and to use. They should be light weight, durable, comfortable, easy to keep clean, and cosmetically acceptable to the patient. Specific instructions should be given the wearer concerning the duration and frequency of its use. Detailed activities should be performed while wearing the splint and during the withdrawal of the splint.

Splints can be classified into three classes—static, semidynamic, and dynamic. Other terms are applicable and other classifications enumerated, but these are the three basic splints to fulfill the following functions.

1. Stabilize (immobilize) joints in a desired position to *rest* the joint, tendons, ligaments, and muscles or maintain a certain bone alignment.
2. Prevent contracture or deformity.
3. Prevent unwanted motion.
4. Gradually stretch contracture to increase range of joint motion.
5. Substitute lost muscle function.
6. Maintain gains achieved by manipulation, corrective surgery, or reconstructive procedures.
7. Relieve pain.

Static splints prevent motion and thus rest the parts indicated. They accomplish this purpose but can also cause disuse atrophy, weakness, stiffness, and dependency. They should never be used longer than is physiologically indicated and should never be used if a dynamic or semidynamic splint is equally effective. Splints should immobilize *only* the intended joints leaving all adjacent joints free to move. Resting splints should have smooth surfaces and be accurately molded to fit properly and to avoid unwanted pressures on boney prominences or nerve areas.

Plaster casts should not be applied circularly but should be laid on in flat slabs, preferably leaving half of the hand uncovered by plaster. When complete enclosure is necessary, the cast should be bivalved as soon as possible.

Semidynamic splints permit no movement but function by positioning the parts to perform at their optimum. For example, the thumb carpometacarpal joint can be splinted in abduction-opposition to facilitate pinch grip with the index finger. Semidynamic splints do not use extrinsic power sources such as rubber bands, springs, and so forth.

Dynamic (functional or kinetic) splints permit movement, guide the movement, prevent unwanted movement, and actively move or resist certain movements. By necessity there is some degree of hinging and some source of power. Intrinsic power utilizes the patient's own muscles whereas extrinsic power uses rubber bands, tension wires, springs, or even electronic or pneumatic units. Dynamic splints are used to overcome gravity, correct muscle imbalance, prevent and correct contracture thus improving range of motion. These splints may offer resistance for active exercise.

Restoration of function by mechanical extrinsically-powered units is still in an experimental stage. Elaborate power units are being constantly developed and engineering technological skills are joining with medical research in this endeavor. These advances are beyond the scope of this text but are well documented by Licht and by Anderson.

Many materials are available for splinting and bracing. Each with specific advocates and each with individual advantages. Currently available are varieties of plaster, plastics, nylon fabrics, and metals for splint construction with instructions from the manufacturers.

Attachment of splints to the hand usually requires straps. These straps should never cross a joint or press against a bony prominence. Areas where nerve pressure is possible should be avoided and a splint should never be so tight or constrictive as to cause edema. Many materials for making straps are also available.

Many splints have been mentioned and illustrated in the preceding chapters for specific conditions and will not be repeated. The following splints are examples of those accepted in current use. It should be repeated that splints must be created to fulfill specific indications after functional evaluation of the hand and determination of the objective of the splint.

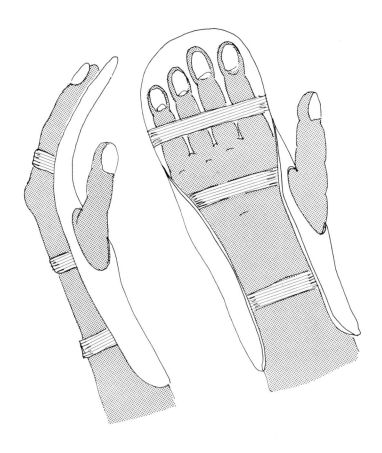

FIGURE 116. Static (rest) splint. This splint can be made of plaster, plastic, Polysar, orthoplast, or other materials and strapped with leather, Velcro, or webbing. It maintains the wrist and fingers in a physiological position. Among its uses are wrist drop from peripheral neuropathies and early flaccid stage of stroke. It prevents deformity, relieves pain, and avoids overstretching of flail musculature.

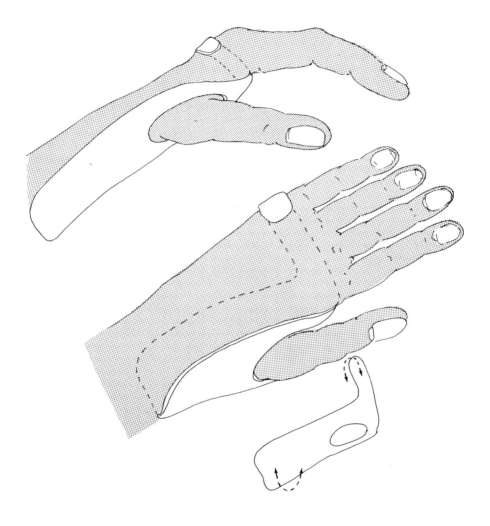

FIGURE 117. Rest wrist splint. This splint can be used as a rest or a semidynamic splint. Its purpose is to maintain the wrist in slight extension yet permit and assist finger and thumb movement. It can be made of any material. It has definite value in treating median nerve compression (carpal tunnel syndrome).

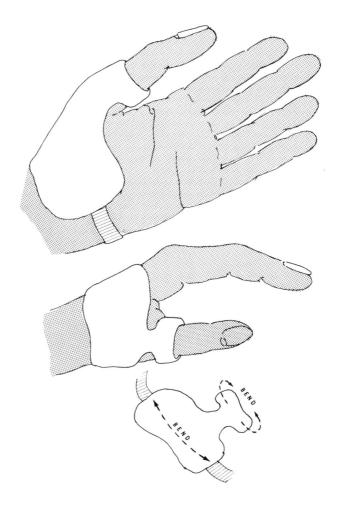

FIGURE 118. Static and semidynamic thumb and splint. Valuable in a flail thumb or in de-generative painful arthritis of carpometacarpal joint. It immobilized the thumb in abduction and opposition permitting tip-to-tip pinch. It has value in spasticity (cerebral palsy), in treating thumb-in-palm, or adducted thumb position.

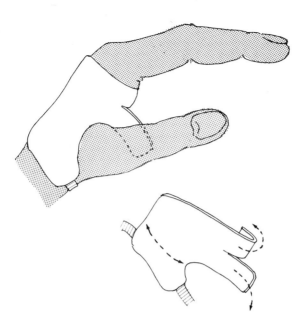

FIGURE 119. Static and semidynamic splint for thumb. This splint mainly maintains thumb in abducted position but does not immobilize the position at the carpometacarpal joint. It may be of value in mild spasticity to decrease thumb-in-palm position.

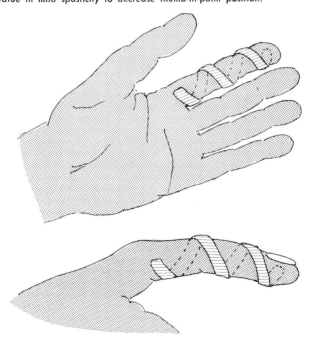

FIGURE 120. Finger rest splint. A simple wrap-around splint is flexible or plastic material used to rest a finger or to maintain gained range of motion in contracture. Restful in post-traumatic or degenerative joint changes.

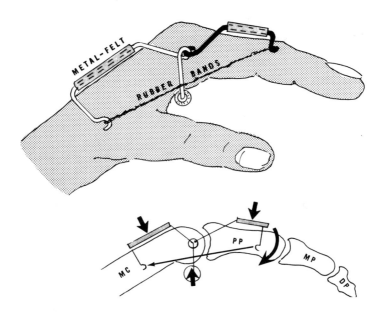

FIGURE 121. Dynamic splint to flex metacarpophalangeal joint, Bunnell knuckle breaker splint. This dynamic splint powered by rubber bands flexes the metacarpophalangeal joint that is contracted following fracture, dislocation, burns, Volkmann's ischemic contracture, and the like. These splints are commercially available.

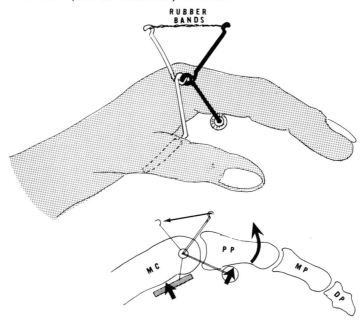

FIGURE 122. Dynamic splint to extend metacarpophalangeal joint(s), reversed Bunnell knuckle breaker. By the power pull of the rubber bands, the proximal phalanx is extended on the metacarpal. There is constant pull while worn. Can be used to exercise and strengthen the proximal flexors.

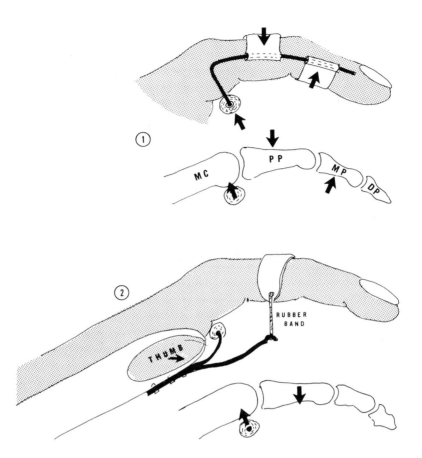

FIGURE 123. Dynamic digit splint. (1) A simple splint made of tensile wire to flex the metacarpophalangeal joint and simultaneously extend the proximal interphalangeal joint. (2) An outrigger extension to a wrist splint to dynamically flex the metacarpophalangeal joint(s). The thumb can be free.

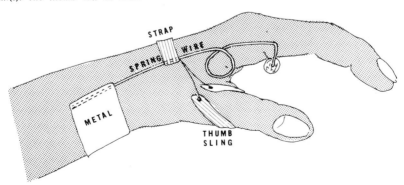

FIGURE 124. Dynamic splint for wrist drop, radial nerve palsy. Using spring wire as power source this simple splint extends the wrist and simultaneously abducts the thumb. Used in radial nerve or nerve root palsies.

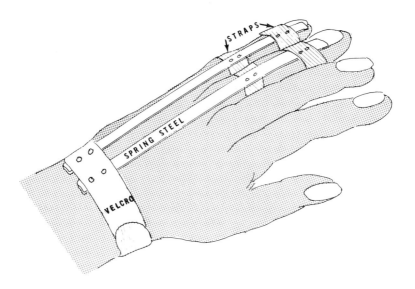

FIGURE 125. Dynamic splint, post-operative in Dupuytren's contracture. Following palmar fasciotomy in Dupuytren's contracture the digital extension can be maintained by the above splint which permits use of the hand keeping the thumb and first two digits free.

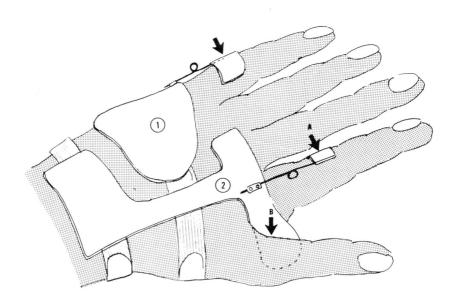

FIGURE 126. Composite dynamic splint, first dorsal interosseous, fifth adduction. Figure shows two splints: (1) spring wire splint to adduct the fifth finger and (2) spring wire splint to assist first dorsal interosseous—index abduction. (B) A flange to abduct the thumb. Usually only one of these splints will be worn or both can be incorporated into one wrist band.

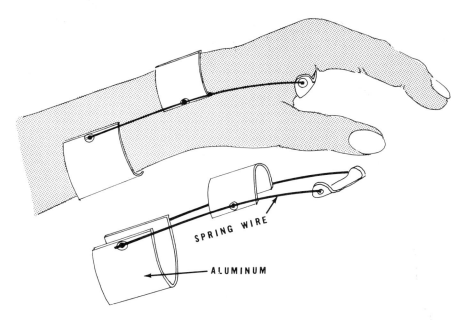

SPRING WIRE

ALUMINUM

FIGURE 127. Dynamic wrist drop splint. This splint can be simply made from spring wire and molded aluminum. It depicts the numerous materials that can be employed in making splints.

BIBLIOGRAPHY

Anderson, M.: Functional Bracing of the Upper Extremities. Charles C Thomas, Publisher, Springfield, Ill., 1958.

Boyes, J. H.: Bunnell's Surgery of the Hand, ed. 4. J. B. Lippincott Company, Philadelphia, 1964.

Bunnell, S.: The Knuckle Bender Splint. U. S. Army Med. Bull., Feb., 1946.

Bunnell, S.: Splinting the Hand. Am. Acad. Ortho. Surg. Instruct., Course Lect., 9:233, 1952.

Licht, S., ed.: Orthotics Etcetera (Physical Medicine Library, Vol. 9). Elizabeth Licht, Publisher, New Haven, Conn., 1966.

Redford, J. B., Gilewich, G., and Jiminez, J.: Simple Splints, Principles and Techniques. University of Alberta Hospital, Canada, 1969.

Wynn Parry, C. B.: Rehabilitation of the Hand. Butterworths, London, 1966.

Index

169